Excel in Health Care

Excel in Health Care

Alan C. Gillies and Phil Baugh

CHAPMAN & HALL MEDICAL
London · Glasgow · Weinheim · New York · Tokyo · Melbourne · Madras

Published by Chapman & Hall, 2–6 Boundary Row, London SE1 8HN, UK

Chapman & Hall, 2–6 Boundary Row, London SE1 8HN, UK

Blackie Academic & Professional, Wester Cleddens Road, Bishopbriggs, Glasgow G64 2NZ, UK

Chapman & Hall GmbH, Pappelallee 3, 69469 Weinheim, Germany

Chapman & Hall USA, One Penn Plaza, 41st Floor, New York NY 10119, USA

Chapman & Hall Japan, ITP-Japan, Kyowa Building, 3F, 2-2-1 Hirakawacho, Chiyoda-ku, Tokyo 102, Japan

Chapman & Hall Australia, Thomas Nelson Australia, 102 Dodds Street, South Melbourne, Victoria 3205, Australia

Chapman & Hall India, R. Seshadri, 32 Second Main Road, CIT East, Madras 600 035, India

First edition 1995

Printed in England by Clays Ltd., St. Ives plc

ISBN 0 412 59760 8

A catalogue record for this book is available from the British Library

∞ Printed on permanent acid-free text paper, manufactured in accordance with ANSI/NISO Z39.48-1992 and ANSI/NISO Z39.48-1984 (Permanence of Paper).

Contents

Preface

Since the advent of the Personal Computer (PC) in the early 1980s, there have been some dramatic changes in the way computers have been employed in business, industry and society at large. The medical profession has also been affected by this revolution in a variety of ways.

At the most hi-tech end of the spectrum, we have witnessed the development of computer tomography which has produced impressive results in terms of clinical diagnosis; intensive care is another area where information technology has played a significant role in aiding the patient monitoring process and helping control patient condition. However, it is also true that computers have become more frequently used throughout medical practice for a variety of purposes.

A decade ago, computer usage in general practice was low. At the time, GPs appeared very sceptical about the possibilities of using computers for keeping patient records. Within general practice, computers were first found to be effective in dealing with repeat prescriptions. Technological developments in processing power and data storage, coupled with some important software developments and the introduction of drug dictionaries and the Read Code Classification have combined to improve facilities immeasurably compared to what was originally available. There has also been a considerable impetus provided by subsidies and grants but, perhaps more importantly, GPs have had to ensure that, with new contractual arrangements, they have been able to claim for all fees and allowances. This in itself encourages greater accuracy in record-keeping and production of appropriate summaries – for which computers are ideal.

It is now routinely possible to store a detailed history for each patient, a record of prescribing, to carry out patient monitoring and surveillance on an individual or collective basis and aid the process of preventative medicine by targeting specific at-risk groups. In addition, with the development of new contractual obligations and fund-holding, it is possible to keep accurate records and produce reports on immunizations and vaccinations, cervical cytology etc. in order to claim the appropriate fees and allowances. Production of a series of standard letters inviting patients for consultation or to clinics also reduces the administrative burden and improves practice support. Developments in computer networking between surgeries and the Family Health Service Authorities will aid in the accuracy of the patient recording process and help in the claiming of allowances. Direct access to waiting list information and other hospital information services will help GPs to make appropriate choices and plan more carefully for their patients' care.

Hospital doctors, particularly consultants and senior registrars involved in research projects and clinical trial analysis, realised early on that computers could aid data manipulation, statistical analysis and graphical presentation of results. Other than this early start, developments in hospital computerization have been slow particularly when compared to other large organizations in business and industry. However, comparison with retail and banking is probably unfair since the procedures involved in all the hospital functions are much more complex. They may be compared better with manufacturing, where developments in computer usage have been much more patchy.

Patient administration systems have been available for some time but have aided doctors little in the patient care process. Information technology has been more successful in the areas of pathology and radiology where procedures can be broken down and results recorded in a straightforward manner. Whilst there have now been developments in hospital information support systems and in case mix management systems, these tend to support the hospital management process rather than patient care. In the next few years, systems will gradually become available which will aid the patient monitoring and care processes.

Whilst these are all important areas, they have involved the development of systems, either by commercial software producers or by the NHS itself, which have involved considerable expenditures. There are a number of ways in which computers coupled with standard commercial software can help the health care process. Packages such as Excel and its forerunners have now been available for over fifteen years in business and industry. Their use by medical personnel and their support staff has, however, been very limited. Spreadsheets with their graphical and statistical add-ins can aid practitioners in a variety of ways. For instance, general practice must not only be capable of recording patient histories, it must also be able to plan and budget for the future. The versatility of spreadsheets can provide a means by which each practice can tailor information technology to its own individual needs. In the case of the development of fund-holding, the increasing demand for devolution of decision-making to the level of those who can make informed decisions requires them to have the necessary technology and procedures to support such a process. This text has been developed to provide GPs and their staff with some of the ideas, concepts and techniques drawn from medical examples.

Introduction: about this book

In writing this book, the authors have drawn on their experience of several years in advising and teaching general practitioners, consultants, practice managers and other medical and related staff about the benefits of using computers in general, and spreadsheets in particular. The purpose of this text is bring together and develop that experience for a greater audience. The text is targeted at medical and related personnel who wish to deepen their experience of using computers in their professional lives.

The text therefore concentrates primarily on the different applications of spreadsheets in the medical environment. In a text of this type it is not possible to cover all the areas within medical practice where spreadsheets can be of use. Rather it is aimed at stimulating interest in a wide range of applications giving the user food for thought in the development of further areas. Neither is the text intended as a replacement for an Excel manual. It does not go into the comprehensive level of detail which a manual will provide. On the other hand it addresses areas of importance which, it is hoped, will maintain the reader's interest and stimulate examination of further points in the manual.

The majority of the text is devoted to an exposition of the functionality within Excel Version 5.0. However, the authors have sought to utilize the functionality of other packages where it is felt that practice applications would benefit from an examination of the ways in which Excel can be integrated with them.

CHAPTER SUMMARY

The chapters have been arranged in a way which takes the user from simpler applications and simple uses of the spreadsheet to more complicated applications and eventually to some of the more complex Excel functions. Each chapter starts with a section called ‘Chapter summary’ which outlines what the chapter is about. The tasks covered are listed in three groups, distinguished by the accompanying bullet characters:

- medical and management tasks covered;
- new Excel functions covered;
- other computing topics covered.

Chapter One commences with an introduction to Windows Version 3.1 and basic movement within Excel Version 5.0. The inclusion of Windows is to ensure good practice within healthcare. Readers already thoroughly familiar with Windows may omit this section but it is particularly recommended for the new user. However, no reader should omit the later section on the accompanying disk.

Chapter Two looks at issues concerned with setting up a simple budgeting system and shows how a spreadsheet can be used to make monthly and annual comparisons. It will deal with simple data entry, the creation of basic formulae, coping and moving data and formatting data for improved presentation. It is completed with an outline of how sheets may be saved for future use and how printed versions can be created.

Chapter Three concentrates on the graphical presentation of the results produced in the previous chapter. It will examine which graphs are suitable for particular purposes including assessment of where 2- and 3-D graphs can be used. With a wide variety of facilities available, emphasis will be given to the process of improving graphs to enhance understanding.

Chapter Four assesses the way in which spreadsheets can be used for performance monitoring. This is demonstrated by taking the example of developmental checks and immunizations for infants. In the process, the database facilities of Excel are examined. This will involve the sorting of and searching for data on specific patients. It will also introduce some of the more complex ways in which Excel can be used to count entries in a patient database.

Chapter Five examines two specific areas. The first involves the use of Excel to develop forecasts of medical expenditure and undertake analysis of possible financial scenarios for a practice. It also addresses the issue of using two of Excel's statistical techniques in the analysis of clinical data in order to estimate associations and relationships

Chapter Six is devoted to examining the problems associated with the optimal use of resources in healthcare in these times of limited budgets. On the principle of only doing the analysis once if possible, it looks at the ways in which these complex tasks may be automated using Excel's macro functions.

Chapter Seven looks at an area of growing importance – medical audit – and shows some of the ways in which the audit process may be automated through the use of Excel functions.

Chapter Eight examines ways in which the results from Excel may be incorporated into a report. The chapter examines the relationship between Excel and Word for Windows in effecting this incorporation and how the process may be developed in such a way as to automate report production over time.

Chapter Nine looks at ways in which disasters may be avoided with a little care and attention. This chapter is not intended to cover issues of trouble-shooting problems encountered with Excel 5.0 for which there is a suitable section in the Excel Manual. Rather it shows the user how to protect the data, spreadsheets and reports which have been produced and how to avoid lost time and effort through judicious use of the facilities available in Excel and Windows. It also deals with other issues such as viruses and the legal constraints on using data.

INSTRUCTIONS

This text is intended to be a workbook enabling the user to learn about Excel's facilities while proceeding through a set of instructions and examples related to healthcare. In order to aid rapid progress we shall follow the convention of indenting all paragraphs which contain instructions. Any such paragraph will commence with either:

🖱 a mouse icon to denote a mouse action.

or:

☛ a pointing hand to denote a keyboard action.

HINTS

At various points in the text, the authors have introduced a 'Hint' box. These boxes are intended to give the user further options in the text. Hints refer to improvements which can be made to the sheet created, short-cuts which can be implemented to speed up the process of using Excel and methods by which problems which are encountered can be circumvented. Excel itself has a feature called TipWizard which will help the user in a number of ways.

HEALTH WARNINGS

The text also includes health warnings which cover a variety of issues from operations the user should or should not carry out through to problems which the user may encounter in the use of the package.

SCREEN IMAGES

The authors have used a variety of screen images in the text to help the user to identify particular points within the text and the corresponding locations in the package. There may, however, be subtle differences resulting from the exact way in which those images were created compared to the way in which the user approaches a problem and which may result from a slightly difference configuration of the application when the machine was first set up. These differences, once allowed for, should not materially affect the sense of the text.

OLDER EQUIPMENT

With the development of computer usage in health care over a number of years, practitioners are using equipment of varying ages. Excel 5.0 has been designed to run on computers containing at least the Intel 80386 chip or later versions. In addition, over the last few years, applications packages have become intense users of computer memory and hard disk space. We recommend that users' computers have a minimum specification of an Intel 80386 processor, 4 megabytes (Mbytes) of memory and an 80 Mbyte hard disk. Users using more packages will need considerably more hard disk capacity.

THE ACCOMPANYING DISK

Accompanying this book is a floppy disk which contains workbooks created in advance to aid instruction. It also contains a selection of workbooks which are partially completed allowing the user to commence reading from intermediate stages. They can also act as templates for your own work. All the workbooks are contained on the floppy disk in a zipped file called 'xlfiles'. Instructions showing the user how to load the workbooks onto the hard disk of the computer are contained in Chapter 1, Section 5.

MICROSOFT OFFICE

Excel is one of a set of applications which are known collectively as the Microsoft Office, which also includes Word for Windows and the presentation package, Powerpoint. With the latest release of Word for Windows (Version 6.0, the next after Version 2.0c!), there is increasing convergence in the ways in which the packages operate which should eventually lead to great improvements in user productivity. Microsoft Office is often the most economical way to obtain Excel, particularly if you use other Microsoft applications.

TRADEMARKS

The following trademarks are acknowledged by the authors as belonging to the Microsoft Corporation:

Microsoft®
Word®
Excel®
Powerpoint®
MS-DOS®
Windows™
Toolbar™
Truetype™

Other trademarks acknowledged are

IBM® and PC®	International Business Machines Corporation
Dbase® and Quattro Pro®	Borland International
Lotus 1-2-3®	Lotus Corporation

Unacknowledged use of any other trademark is entirely unintentional and will be happily acknowledged by the authors in any future edition if notified.

1

The computer arrives: how to start

1.1 CHAPTER SUMMARY

You now have a brand new computer on your desk. What can you do with it? Half your colleagues tell you it will be the best thing that ever happened to you, the other will tell you it's a disaster. Hopefully, someone will tell you how to switch it on...

This chapter will tell you:

- what all the bits of the computer do;
- how to get started with the hardware and software;
- about your computer;
- about Windows 3.1;
- what Excel (version 5) looks like;
- how to move around in Excel;
- how to identify or 'paint' areas of the sheet.

1.2 GETTING STARTED

One of the hardest tasks with any computer is getting started: the initial learning curve can be very steep, as shown in Fig. 1.1.

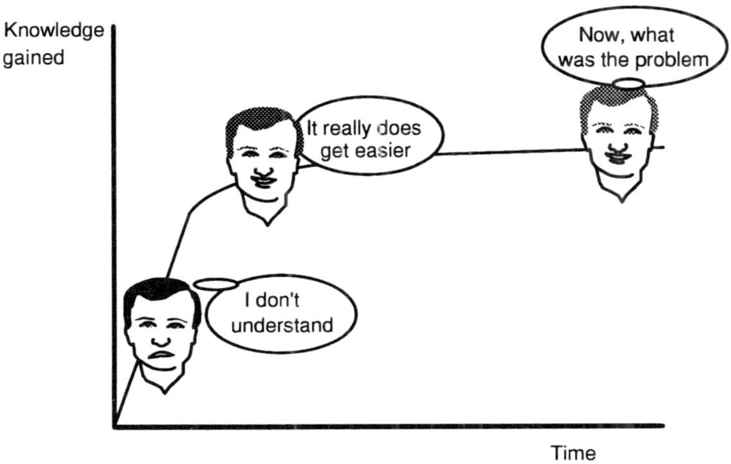
Knowledge gained
Now, what was the problem
It really does get easier
I don't understand
Time

Fig. 1.1 The learning curve.

First, we have to find the on/off switch, usually either on the front panel or round the side. Switch on and the system comes to life – the computer will 'boot up'. This involves the computer loading a special program called the operating system into memory and testing that it can find all the required parts. We shall start by considering all the components of the system by going on a guided tour of the PC.

1.3 A GUIDED TOUR OF THE PC

A PC (Personal Computer) is a computer system, consists of several components that work together, principally the *monitor*, the *system unit,* and the *keyboard*. In addition there may be other pieces of equipment linked to the system, such as printers, plotters and modems. These are called *peripherals*.

The monitor is a cathode ray tube, similar to that in a television. Monochrome monitors are suitable for word-processing or spreadsheeting, colour monitors are much better for graphics. Picture definition, i.e. the standard of resolution, can be very high and quality is constantly improving. The current modern standards are VGA (Video

Graphics Array) and Super VGA (Super Video Graphics Array) - used on some machines and giving a better definition.

1.3.1 System unit

The *system unit* is the part of the system which manipulates the information. Within the metal case are circuit boards on which are mounted a number of microprocessors. The most important of these is the CPU (Central Processing Unit), which is the 'brain' of the PC. The companies which manufacture PC microprocessors (principally Intel) are constantly improving them, so PCs are becoming more and more powerful. The original IBM PC contained the Intel 8088 chip. The IBM AT contained the Intel 80286 and the PS/2 the 80386 - each microprocessor more powerful than its predecessor in terms of number of instructions per second which are performed. The latest PCs have even faster processors, usually 80486 or 486s. These are needed to handle the demands of the latest generation of Windows packages, which are very resource intensive. Intel has recently introduced the Pentium chip which promises faster processing still. Other manufacturers, e.g. IBM, Cyrix are starting to produce their own competing processors.

The circuit board also holds the memory chips (basic memory comprises 640 Kilobytes (Kbytes) in total - around 640,000 keyboard characters of data) available to store the programs and data employed in a particular application. These memory chips are called Dynamic RAM (random access memory) – once the power supply is switched off programs and data are lost. The resource intensity of modern machines together with user demands means that 640 Kbytes is insufficient. Most modern PCs come with memory expanded up to 4 or even 8 Mbytes and the potential for much more.

In addition, computers need a means of long-term storage. The system unit contains a *fixed disk,* used for long-term storage of programs and data. Fixed disks are contained in a hermetically sealed unit so that particles of dust, smoke or moisture cannot harm them. They spin at over 3000 revolutions per minute enabling rapid data access and can store a great deal of data typically between 20 Mbytes and 400 Mbytes – approximately 20 to 400 million characters of information.

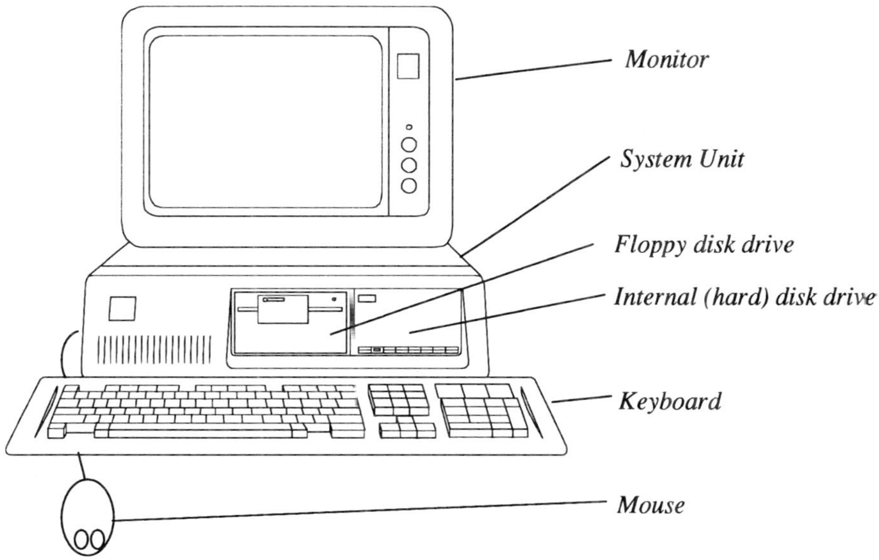

Fig. 1.2 The PC.

Since there is a need to get the programs and personal data into the machine in the first place a *floppy disk* is required - This is a flexible plastic disk with a magnetic coating and comes in two sizes – $3^1/_2$ inch diameter or $5^1/_4$ inch diameter. It can typically hold from 360Kbytes (around 360,000 keyboard characters of information) to 1.44 Mbytes of data. To prevent the disk being damaged, it is kept within a stiff card or plastic cover, resulting in only a small area of the surface being exposed. Since disks can be used with a wide variety of incompatible computers, it is necessary to format any disk (fixed or floppy) for the computer with which it is to be used (see below). The $3^1/_2$ inch disks are more commonly used because they are smaller, more robust and hold more data. The different types of disk are compared in Table 1.1.

Optical storage of information represents the way forward in many applications where there is a requirement for large amounts of data to be kept over long periods. Patient records is one area where such storage will be necessary in the long-term since detailed data must be kept on a patient over his or her lifetime. This aspect of data storage in the practice is yet to be fully explored by doctors or practice managers.

Table 1.1 Comparison of Floppy disk types

	3.5 in disks	*5.25in disks*
Appearance	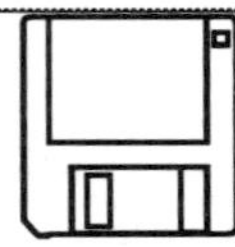	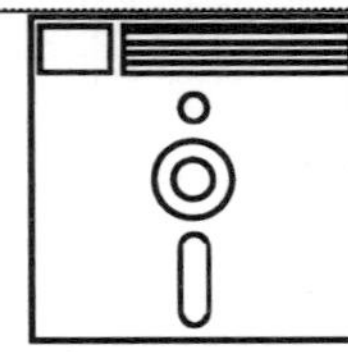
Physical characteristics	Robust; in rigid protective case	Relatively fragile
Size	More compact	Less compact
Data storage	Storage 720k - 1.44 Mb	Storage 360k - 1.2Mb
Reliability at maximum density	High Density (HD) mode very reliable	HD mode less reliable

The *keyboard* is the major input device for the PC i.e. the means through which people can interact with the computer and the programs running on it. The central area is the familiar (to those of you who can type!!) QWERTY keyboard. There are also many other keys which we will explore as the book unfolds.

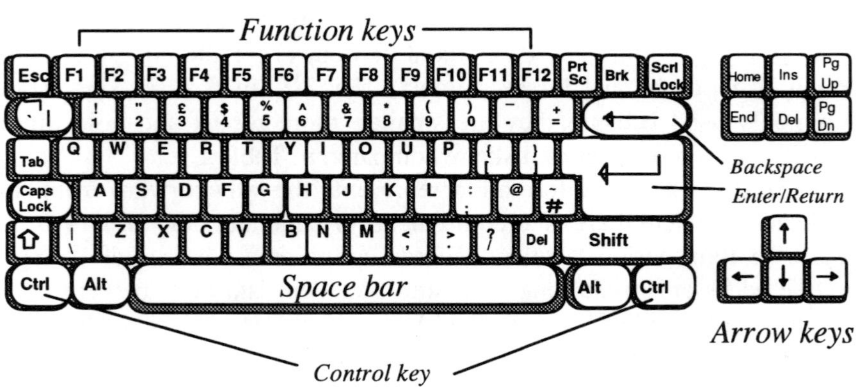

Fig. 1.3 A typical keyboard.

Keyboards may differ from PC to PC: standards are only beginning to emerge in terms of number of keys and their position.

1.3.2 Mouse

The *mouse* has also become a common input device, which, when coupled with a Windows environment, improves the speed with which commands can be given to the computer and opens up use of the computer especially to those who have limited keyboard skills or who do not need extensive typing skills. There are two main types of mice, two-button and three-button:

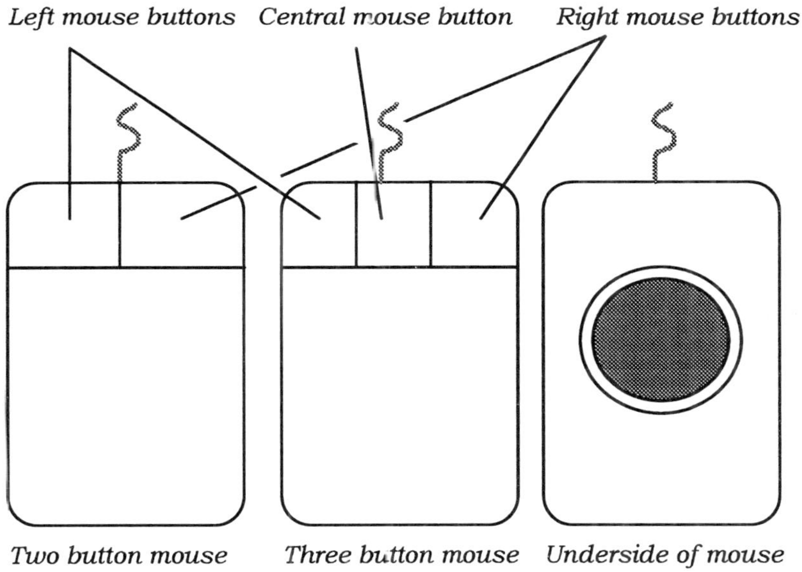

Fig. 1.4 The mouse.

The principal buttons are positioned on the left and right of the mouse. The centre button, if available, is not used. In this book, we shall assume that, when asked to press a button on the mouse, it is the left button unless specifically stated. Underneath the mouse is a rolling ball which detects movement as the mouse is moved. Do not touch this as grease from your fingers will collect dust and may reduce the mouse's effectiveness. There are a number of actions which need to be mastered with the mouse, (Table 1.2):

Table 1.2 Mouse actions

Action	*Explanation*
Move	requires you to move the whole mouse around physically on the desk. The action will be mimicked on the screen.
Click	requires you to press once on the left hand button of the mouse to highlight a specific object or cell.
Right-Click	requires you to press once on the right hand button of the mouse to highlight a specific object or cell.
Select	requires you to press once on the left hand button of the mouse to select an item from a menu or list.
Double-click	requires you to press twice in quick succession (almost like an involuntary twitch!) on the left hand button of the mouse without moving the mouse in between.
Drag	requires you to move to an object, press down the left hand button of the mouse and without releasing the button, move the mouse to the location required on the screen. Once at the destination, release the mouse button. This operation is used to 'paint' areas in Excel as we shall see later.

1.4 USING THE WINDOWS ENVIRONMENT

1.4.1 Windows (version 3.1)

Unlike MS-DOS™ which was developed in the 1970s, an era in which information was displayed in a predominantly text-based manner, WINDOWS™ (hereafter simply referred to as Windows) uses the richer graphical environment developed in the 1980s. Windows makes full use of what is known as WIMPs: windows, icons, mice and pointers. The screen should be viewed as a desk-top. Work currently on the desktop is displayed in windows. The windows can be re-arranged on the desktop in much the same way as papers and files can be re-arranged on a desk. Items not currently open on the desktop may be shown as icons. These are small images which indicate the availability of items and display their type by the particular item in use.

An essential item for ease of use of a windows environment is the mouse described earlier, which can drive a variety of pointers (principally arrows and crosses) around the screen. The use of the mouse and the associated screen pointer facilitates the selection of items from pop-up and pull-down menus.

The most important features of Windows is its standardization in that many if not most of the commands learnt for one application will operate in exactly the same way for another. This reduces learning time for any one application considerably and allows one to 'guess' how many of the operations in an application might work from the experience of another. If you are already familiar with Word for Windows then many of the operations in Excel will in part already be familiar to you. For example using Cut and Paste in Edit is the same in Excel and Word for Windows. It also means that, if you are using a Windows application for the first time then, having followed this text, you should be well on the way to understanding other Windows applications.

The next section provides an introduction to the Windows environment, based around the Program Manager. If you are familiar with this already, you may proceed to section 1.5 without missing anything.

1.4.2 The Program Manager

If you are not already within windows, but are facing a DOS prompt:

☛ **Type** WIN↵ (↵ is the [Return] or [Enter] key) .

After a few seconds, the Windows desktop will appear. The first application that you see will be the Program Manager. The elements of the desktop are described below, and a sample desktop shown in Fig.1.5.

🖰 **Click** on ⊟ (This is the Control Menu Box in the top left corner).

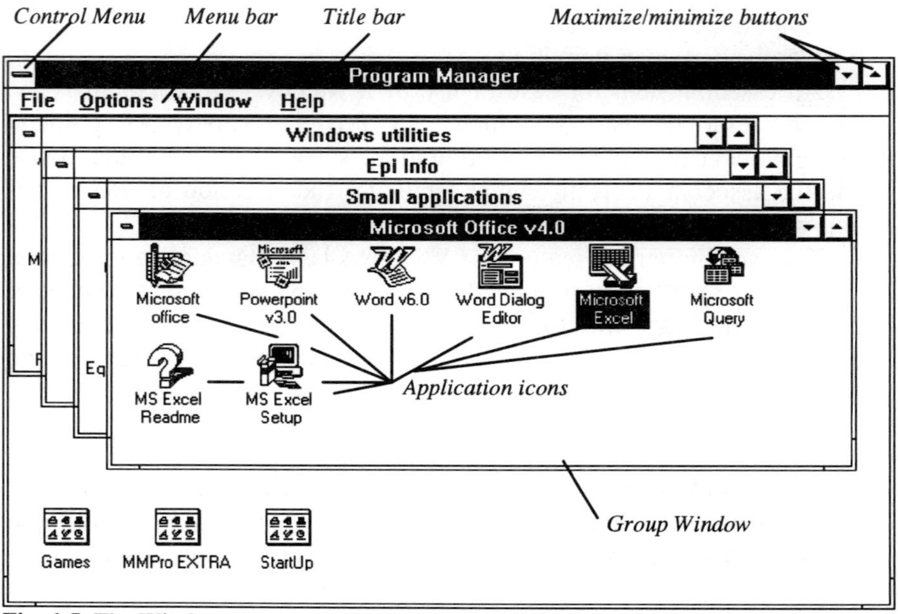

Fig. 1.5 The Windows Program Manager.

The control menu will appear. Each of the items in the box can be selected. Those which are shown as feint are not currently available. In the case of these items, they can all be obtained through use of the mouse without opening the control box.

Click on ▭ again to close down the menu.

The title bar shows the name of an application, e.g. Program Manager. If there is more than one window open, the active window will be shown with a different colour or in greater colour intensity. The title is the name of an application or a document used in that window.

Click on the word 'File' in the menu bar.

The file menu, shown in Fig. 1.6, will appear. Items not currently available will be shown in feint. Click on any part of the window other than the menu to close the current menu.

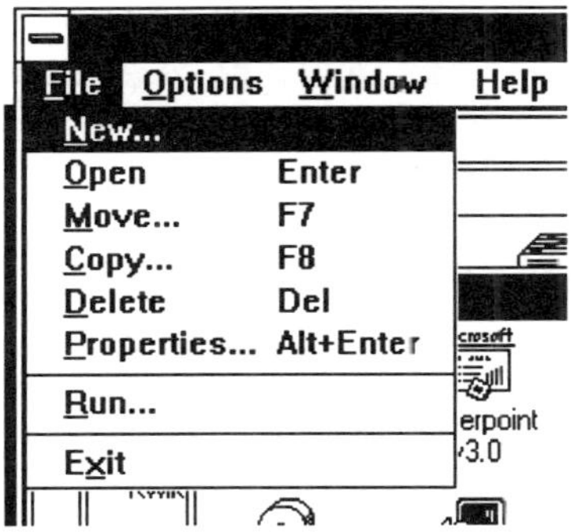

Fig. 1.6 File menu from Program Manager.

If a window is not large enough to contain all the information required, then it will have scroll bars to enable movement to different parts of a document which may not be currently displayed on the screen:

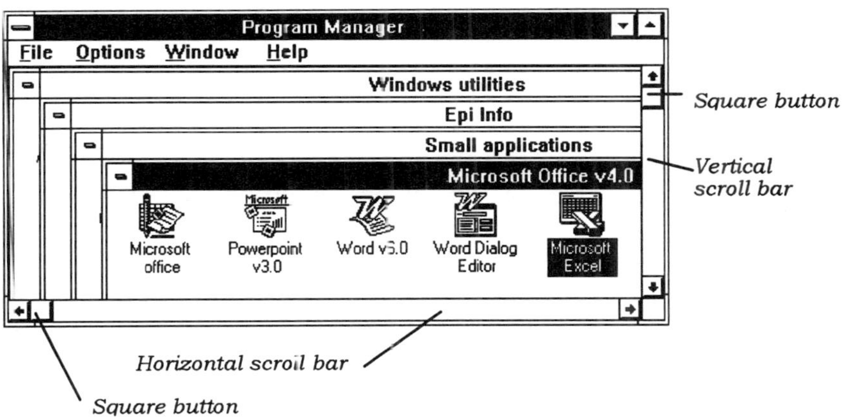

Fig. 1.7 Scroll bars.

To move vertically,

- **Click** and **hold down** the mouse button with the pointer resting on the square button in the vertical scroll bar.
- **Drag** it down the bar – as you drag, the button or sometimes just an outline moves with you.

Release the button at an appropriate point. Use the same procedure for the horizontal bar. Use this manoeuvre to practise getting used to the dragging action of the mouse.

In the top right corner are the Maximize and Minimize buttons:

- **Click** on the (Maximize button) to allow the window to fill the screen.

A Restore button will now appear.

- **Click** on (the Restore button) to restore the window to its previous size.
- **Click** on (the Minimize button) to reduce the Window to an icon:
- **Double-click** on the icon to restore the Window. Don't worry if it takes a few attempts to master the double-click; it is one of the trickier actions with the mouse. The commonest problem is holding the mouse still between clicks. If at first you don't succeed, keep trying, it gets easier!

The window can be re-sized by dragging the sides or corners of the window. To re-size a window:

- **Move** to a border (a double-headed arrow or will appear).
- **Drag** the mouse (remember that dragging means holding down the left mouse button whilst the mouse is moved) until the box is the correct size and release. At first an outline will move with the double headed arrow. Then a single outline will appear.

1.4.3 File Manager

It is not our intention to deal with many aspects of Windows here since the text is primarily concerned with Excel but File Manager is a useful tool to understand for the best use of Excel later on. You may like to return to this section when you have read the next section about Excel itself. File Manager offers an alternative means of using many of the DOS commands associated with the management of files in a friendlier environment. It also offers a number of facilities which are not directly available at DOS level.

You should find the File Manager within the Program Manager – most likely in Main or possibly Accessories depending on how the Program Manager has been set up. Look for the icon below:

Hint: It's yellow!

Double-click on 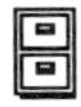.

The first thing to note is that the File Manager screen has many elements we have seen before: name bar, menu bar, control menu button, Maximize/Minimize buttons, scroll bars. This is because in Windows, all applications have a similar appearance and the same general features. The window which appears will depend upon the directory in which you are currently located. Fig. 1.8 assumes that you are in the Excel directory.

Hint: If you want to go to the Excel directory, find 'excel' in the directory tree and click on it.

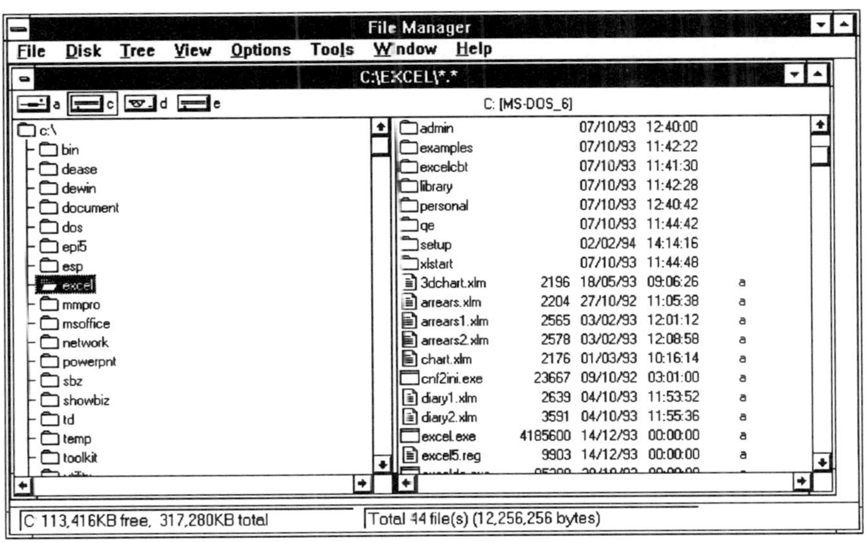

Fig. 1.8 The Windows File Manager.

Now we shall consider some of the basic operations of the File Manager:

a) Formatting a disk

Magnetic disks generally come as standard to be used on a wide variety of different computers. However, each operating system has a different way of addressing the disk which means that the floppy disk used on an IBM-compatible PC cannot be read by an Apple Macintosh without special software. When a disk is first purchased it must be formatted to the requirements of the operating system of the machine with which it is to be used. The procedure is as follows:

- **Insert** a new floppy disk in Drive A:
- **Select** 'Disk'.
- **Select** 'Format Disk'.
- **Click** on [OK].
- **Click** on [Yes].

Health Warning: When the computer puts up a message in a box or asks you to confirm an action, the authors refer to this as a 'Have you lost your presence of mind?' box. Whatever form this takes, always be sure to take a deep breath and think before you proceed....

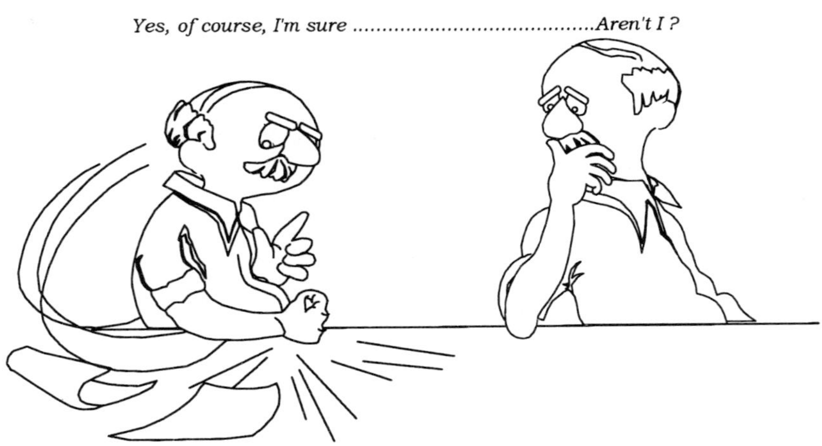

b) Formatting a system disk

Occasionally it will be necessary to format a disk putting the system files on it. The system files contain the DOS commands necessary for 'booting' the system. These are not required when using a machine with hard disk since the hard disk holds the system files. They are, however, required if a machine with floppy disks only is used. To produce a system disk:

- **Select** 'Disk'.
- **Select** 'Make System Disk'.
- **Click** on Yes (Sure about copying system files onto disk).

> **Health Warning:** Do **NOT** re-format a disk on which you already have data. The data will be erased!

c) Labelling the disk

If you have an untidy desk, a computer will not help you – you will have untidy files and disks. However, there are ways in which the computer can help with organization. We can label disks logically, i.e. on the disk itself, as well as physically:

- **Select** 'Disk'.
- **Select** 'Label Disk'.
- **Type** a name for the disk (no longer than 8 characters).
- **Click** on OK.

Hint: It is useful if the logical name put on the disk is the same as the one you write on the front cover! Note that a label may be attached at the formatting stage.

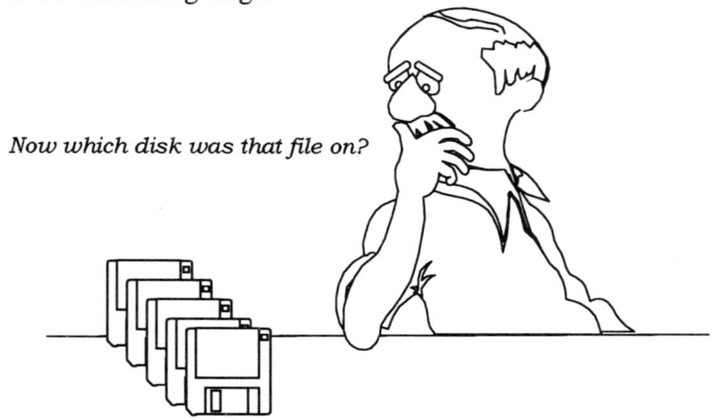

d) Creating directories

The developers of Windows and indeed, the operating systems which preceded it have tried to fashion the keeping of files in the same way one would keep paper files within an office. The files on the disk can be organized into directories which correspond to the drawers in a filing cabinet. Files may be put into each directory as they would be put in the drawers if they were paper files.

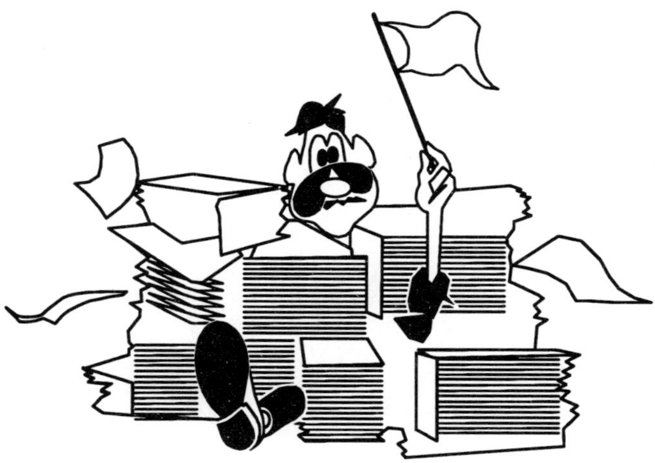

Fig. 1.9 'Computers are no substitute for a tidy mind.'

However, it is likely that if your patient records are in a mess then your computer files will be as well. Computers may help in organizing your work but they cannot turn a bad filing system into a good one. To create a new directory:

- **Click** on c in the bar at the top of the window.
- **Click** on c:\ (unless it is already highlighted)
- **Select** 'File' from the menu bar.
- **Select** 'Create Directory'.
- **Type** FHSA *(this is the name of our directory).*

It is also possible to create sub-directories within each directory (and sub-sub-directories). The directory where sub-directories are to be placed must first be highlighted:

- **Select** 'FHSA' directory.
- **Select** 'File' from the menu bar.
- **Select** 'Create Directory'.
- **Type** the name of a directory e.g. FHSADATA.
- **Click** on OK.

The end result should look like:

e) Copying a File

The copying process in Windows is more versatile than with DOS although it does take a little time to get used to and offers little benefit for copying an individual file. Firstly we need to see the files which we are going to copy:

- **Double-click** on c:\

The tree structure of the directory will appear if not already showing. Double-click switches the tree structure display on and off.

- **Click** on 'EXCEL' Directory.
- **Click** on 'FHSA.XLS' in the Excel window (the file will be highlighted).

☛ **Hold down** the [Ctrl] key and **hold down** the left button on the file - a file icon will appear as you move the mouse.

🖱 **Drag** the icon to the FHSA directory.

Release the mouse button first, then the [Ctrl] key.

🖱 **Click** on [Yes] to confirm the mouse action and copy the file.

This is another example of a 'have you lost your presence of mind?' box, used this time to confirm the copying action.

> **Hint**: The [Ctrl] key is not needed if the file is copied from one disk to another, e.g from the floppy drive to the hard disk. Without the [Ctrl] key in our example, we would move the file from one directory to another on the same disk.

f) Copying consecutive files

There are two distinct ways to copy more than one file depending on whether the files appear consecutively on the screen or not. If they do:

🖱 **Click** on 'EXCEL' Directory.

🖱 **Click** on a file in the Excel directory Window.

☛ **Hold down** the [⇧] key – this is the Shift key.

🖱 **Click** on a file below the highlighted file in the listing (all intervening files will be highlighted).

☛ **Hold down** the [Ctrl] key and

🖱 **hold down** the left button on the highlighted area.

🖱 **Drag** the icon to the FHSA directory and release.

🖱 **Click** on [Yes] to complete the copying procedure.

g) Copying non-consecutive files

If the files are not listed consecutively:

🖱 **Click** on 'EXCEL' Directory.

☛ **Hold down** the [Ctrl] key.

🖱 **Click** on three separate files in the list.

🖱 **Hold down** the left button on the last highlighted area.

Drag the icon to the FHSA directory and release.

Note that this time you are prompted to ask you if you wish to overwrite the existing files if they already been copied.

Click on [Yes] to complete the copying procedure.

h) Moving files

It is possible in the most recent versions of DOS (6.0 and later) to move files from one directory to another although in earlier versions it is not. This facility is available in File Manager as well. In effect moving files involves copying to the destination directory and deleting in the source directory):

Click on 'EXCEL' directory.

Click on another file.

Hold down the left mouse button and **drag** the file to the FHSA directory.

Click on [Yes] to confirm moving the files.

Note that the files have been removed from the source directory. Now use the same process to return the file to the EXCEL directory

i) Deleting files

Files can be deleted from the disk again using the option to remove several files of different types:

Click on 'FHSA' directory .

Click on the first file.

☛ **Hold down** the [⇧] key

Click on the last file.

Select 'File' from the menu bar.

Select 'Delete'.

Click on [OK].

Confirmation of the file to be removed will be requested on each occasion unless this protection has been removed by changing the protection options. This is not recommended as it amounts to short-circuiting a 'have you lost your presence of mind' message.

Alternatively, a keyboard shortcut can be used:

Highlight the files to be deleted.

Press the [Delete] or [Del] key.

Click on OK.

You can delete whole directories with or without sub-directories.

Click on 'FHSA' directory.

Press the [Delete] or [Del] key.

Click on OK.

Note that you are prompted both times to try to prevent too much damage!

j) Renaming files

It is useful sometimes to rename files in order to free existing names for other purposes.

Click on 'EXCEL' directory.

Click on a file.

Select 'File' from the menu bar.

Select 'Rename'.

Type in a new name for the file: 'RENAMED.DOC'.

Click on OK.

Renaming only changes the name of the file, not the contents.

Now please close the File Manager by

Select 'File' from the menu bar.

Select 'Exit' to return to the Program Manager.

Hint: A quick way to close down any window is to

Double-click on .

Essentially using a mouse is no more difficult than steering a car. However for first-time users, it can appear quite difficult. Just as a new driver steering a car tends to make exaggerated movements, so all that is required with the mouse is a light touch. Some people manage to master neither car or mouse! For those who need further practice in a non-serious environment then try a game:

Select 'Window' from the main menu .

Select 'Games' in the lower half of the menu.

Click on 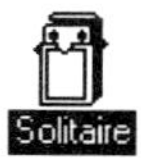

.

Hint: It is possible if you cannot find the Solitaire icon that someone has moved or deleted it to prevent such a frivolous activity. We shall however, use it for a serious purpose.

You are now presented with the classic card game of patience or solitaire:

- Move cards around by **dragging** with the mouse.
- Turn over the cards by **clicking** on the card back (or green circle at the end of the pile).

This is an excellent way to familiarize yourself with the Windows environment and the actions of the mouse. It comes highly recommended but is best done out of office hours.

When finished:

Select 'Game' from the menu bar.

Select 'Exit' to return to the Program Manager.

1.5 THE DISK ACCOMPANYING THIS BOOK

Health Warning:	This section is essential if you wish to use the later examples in this book.

Before proceeding further, you need to copy the files from the accompanying disk into your Excel working directory. Place the floppy disk in your floppy disk drive and return to the Windows file manager:

Select 'Window' from the menu bar.

Select 'Main' from lower half of the menu (unless File Manager has been moved to another group).

Double-click on 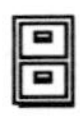

Select 'File' from the menu bar

Select 'Run'

☞ **Type** a:\xlfiles↵

The computer should now extract the files from the floppy disk and place them in your Excel directory.

If version 5.0 of Excel is unavailable, then you may be able to work through many of the examples using Excel 4.0. For this purpose, a set of files is included in Excel 4.0 format. To extract these instead:

Click on ├ excel

Select 'File' from the menu bar

Select 'Run'

☞ **Type** a:\xl4files↵

Unfortunately, there have been considerable changes between versions 4.0 and 5.0, particularly in the interface (i.e. the way in which you give instructions to the computer). Therefore, it is strongly advised that you follow the examples with version 5.0 where possible. A full list of the differences between versions is given in the appendix at the end of the book.

In particular, a novice user of Excel is not advised to try to follow this book with version 4.0 and is strongly advised to purchase the upgrade to version 5.0. This is relatively expensive if acquired through the commercial market; it may be acquired more cheaply through a local University if you are part of a teaching department, or through a health authority purchasing agreement.

1.6 MICROSOFT EXCEL (VERSION 5.0)

The spreadsheet is probably the most versatile piece of PC software available. 'Visicalc', the first spreadsheet, is recognised as having been a major factor in causing the micro-computer revolution in the late 1970s and early 1980s. Essentially a spreadsheet is an electronic piece of paper divided into rows and columns. The intersection of a row and column forms a cell.

Each cell is identified by the row and column that it occupies:

	A	B	C
1	*cell A1*	*cell B1*	*cell C1*
2	*cell A2*	*cell B2*	*cell C2*
3	*cell A3*	*cell B3*	*cell C3*

Fig. 1.10 Schematic representation of rows, columns and cells.

Unlike a piece of paper, each cell can contain more than just text or a number, most importantly it can contain a formula detailing how the value displayed in that cell is to be calculated. Excel is one of a new generation of spreadsheets that not only has the formulas, graphics and data manipulation capabilities of earlier spreadsheets such as the first version of Lotus 1-2-3, but includes many superior facilities for formatting the spreadsheet to improve presentation. The latest version of Excel, version 5.0 offers lots of shortcuts and easier ways to carry out common tasks.

Excel operates in the Windows environment making full use of windows, icons, the mouse and pointers. It is controlled largely by using the mouse to point at objects and 'clicking' the mouse to activate the object, rather than typing in commands.

As planning and budgeting are going to become an increasingly important part of practice activities, Excel is an excellent tool to aid the management of cash-limited budgets and other financial planning activities.

To start Excel from the Windows environment,

Double-click on 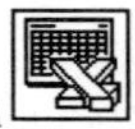 the Excel spreadsheet icon

which is generally found either in a group of its own or in the Windows Applications group. The spreadsheet will now be loaded. Please note, we have omitted the grid lines from the sheet in the interests of clarity.

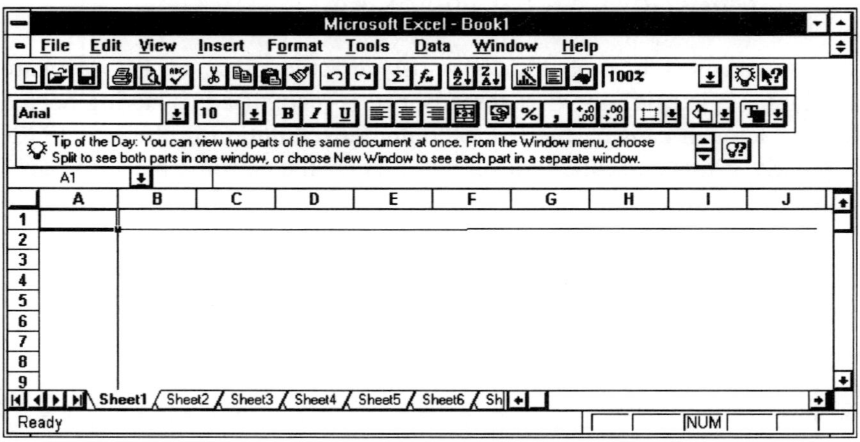

Fig. 1.11 Excel version 5.0: opening screen

There are many features of the Windows environment here that are common to the Windows applications that we have already seen, but there are some new ones as well.

1.6.1 The toolbars

Excel (particularly version 4.0 upwards) makes extensive use of toolbars. These are a set of 'buttons' which, when clicked on, perform an operation. They provide shortcuts to a number of standard operations.

Excel version 5.0 has no less than 13 toolbars to cover function such as drawing, macros, charting and so on.

At this stage we shall start with the main toolbar that appears on our opening screen:

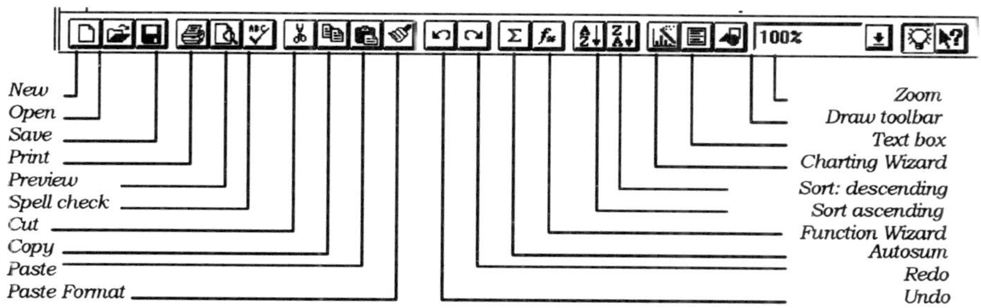

Fig. 1.12 The main toolbar.

Rather than give you indigestion at this point, we shall delay explanation of each function until later in the text. The toolbar is simply a shortcut way of entering commands into the computer.

For example,

Click on the  button.

This has the same effect as

Select 'File' from the menu bar.

Select 'New' from the 'File' menu.

In fact the above is just one of several toolbars which are designed to help us use Excel more quickly and easily. In what follows we shall make use of the toolbars as much as possible. However, many of them are not available in earlier versions (see the Appendix for details)

If you're not sure which button does what then simply move the mouse so that the pointer on the screen lies over the required toolbar button. After a short pause, a message will appear:

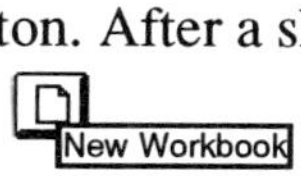

a) Vertical/horizontal movement

This works in a similar way to other Windows applications, e.g. the Program Manager that you have already seen. Place the arrow in the scroll bar and click on the square down arrow screen button to achieve single cell movement, or hold down for multi-cell movement. To move selectively up or down (right or left), hold the left mouse button down on the scroll bar button (i.e. the blank button which is situated within the scroll bar) and drag it gently down the bar (or rightward along the bar). Notice the highlight (the faint square outline) move. When the mouse button is released the scroll button will move to the highlight and movement in the spreadsheet will be effected.

b) Highlighting areas (painting the screen)

Highlighting areas of the sheet to work with them is known as painting. This is a fundamental operation which will allow us to copy, move, format or otherwise edit areas of the sheet.

Take the blank sheet on the screen in front of you.

🖱 Place the arrow in cell B3, **hold down** the left-hand button and 'drag' the mouse across the sheet to cell F8.

Hint: Later in the text, we shall simply record this instruction as:

☛ **Paint** B3 to F8.

The end result of painting this region of the sheet is shown in Fig. 1.13.

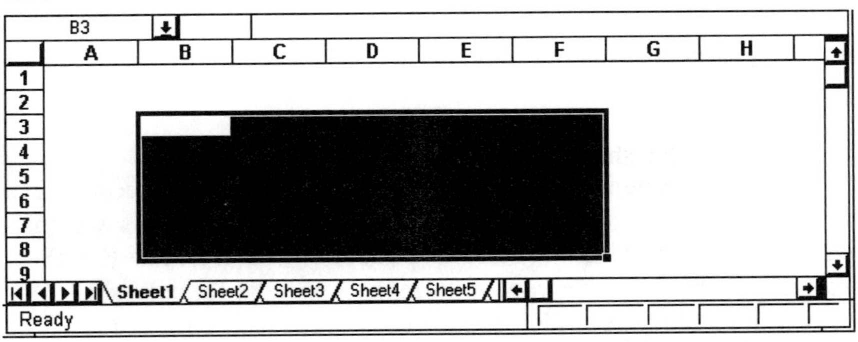

Fig. 1.13 Empty sheet with painted area from B3 to F8.

To extend the painted area:

☛ **Hold down** the [⇧] key and the left mouse button simultaneously and **drag** the mouse across the tabletop to cell H8 and release.

There should now be a painted area extending from B3 down to H8.

Alternatively, you may wish to paint two or more separate areas. This commonly occurs when you wish to select data together with labels. For example, to paint the areas B3 to F3 and B5 to F8:

- **Paint** the cells B3 to F3, as above.
- **Hold down** the [Ctrl] key and **click** on B5.
- **Hold down** the left mouse button simultaneously and
- **Drag** the mouse across the tabletop to cell F8 and release. .

There should now be two painted areas extending from B3 to F3 and down from B5 to F8.

c) Moving in painted areas:

Pressing the ⇥ or ↵ key moves you through cells in painted area:

- **Press** ⇥ for horizontal movement .
- **Press** ↵ for vertical movement.

d) Selecting the entire sheet

You can paint the entire sheet by selecting the square grey button at the top left hand corner of the sheet:

- **Click** on 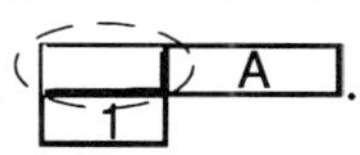.

1.6.2 Tabs

At the bottom of the sheet is a set of tabs, illustrated in Fig. 1.14

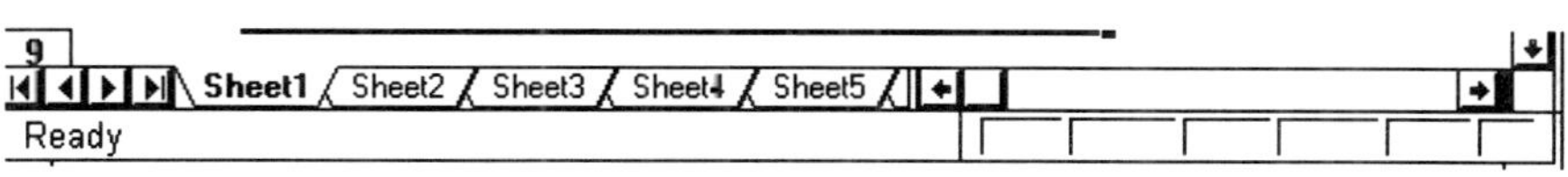

Fig.1.14 The tabs displayed at the bottom of the sheet.

The sheet you see is simply the first of a large number available to you. A typical use of this facility might involve annual data on prescribing costs. On the top sheet one would have data relating to the current year. On the sheets beneath, one could have data from previous years. This would allow comparison over time. This facility is often referred to as using multidimensional spreadsheets. In such a case, time becomes the third dimension:

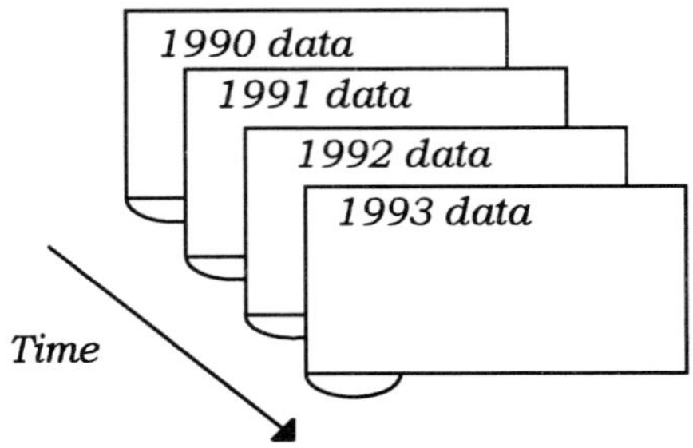

Fig.1.15 Use of tabs in multidimensional spreadsheets (schematic).

Previous versions of Excel have not had this feature, although there was a feature called Workbooks which did similar things in a more limited way. We shall demonstrate this facility later in the book.

1.6.3 The pointers

The pointer that appears on the screen in Excel is context dependent. The commonest pointer when working in an Excel sheet is an outlined cross:

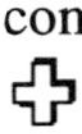

However, other pointers are used in different contexts and we shall explain them as we encounter them. The different pointers may appear confusing at first, but can be extremely helpful once their meaning is grasped.

2

Setting up a simple budget

2.1 CHAPTER SUMMARY

In these days of increased responsibility for budgetary control, one of the most crucial tasks is ensuring that actual spending does not exceed the planned budget. This chapter shows how to use a spreadsheet to compare the figures on a monthly and annual basis.

We will introduce a simple spreadsheet to enable

- annual and monthly expenditure to be tracked;
- planned and actual budgets to be compared.

In the process we shall introduce the following features of Excel:

- data entry;
- copying and moving data within the sheet;
- Autofill;
- pre-defined functions, and the Autosum facility;
- formatting: data types, fonts, presentation;
- saving and printing the sheet.

2.2 MANAGING THE PRACTICE BUDGET

It was stated earlier that spreadsheets had been primarily responsible for the early development of the use of microcomputers in business. The principal reason was the versatility of spreadsheets in the development of financial plans and budgets allowing for the easy manipulation of fairly complex calculations. For this use, the spreadsheet is ideal. However, as we shall see later, modern spreadsheets are not limited solely to numerical calculations but can be used to tackle a wide variety of business and industrial problems.
As an example of the way in which we can use Excel within the practice we shall set up a practice budget showing the planned expenditure and actual expenditure over a twelve month period. The variance of actual from planned expenditure will be shown, as well as annual totals.

2.2.1 Opening a sheet

Firstly a data sheet on file will be brought on screen. We shall use the toolbar button which is found near the top left-hand corner of the screen:

Click on .

As an alternative we could use the following:

Select 'File' from the menu bar.

The file menu, shown in Fig. 2.1, gives us a whole series of options to do with file and print management.

Select 'Open'.

This illustrates a general feature of Excel, that the toolbars provide a quick method, but using the menus gives maximum flexibility. Whichever method we use, we are now presented with a dialog box shown in Fig. 2.2.

Select 'budget.xls' from the menu of files.

Click on OK.

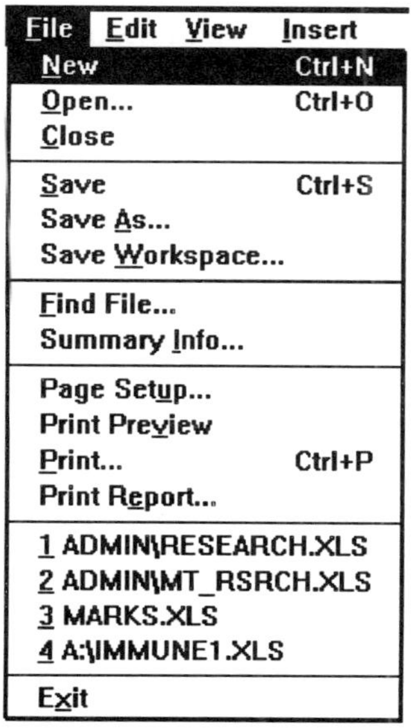

Fig 2.1 The file menu.

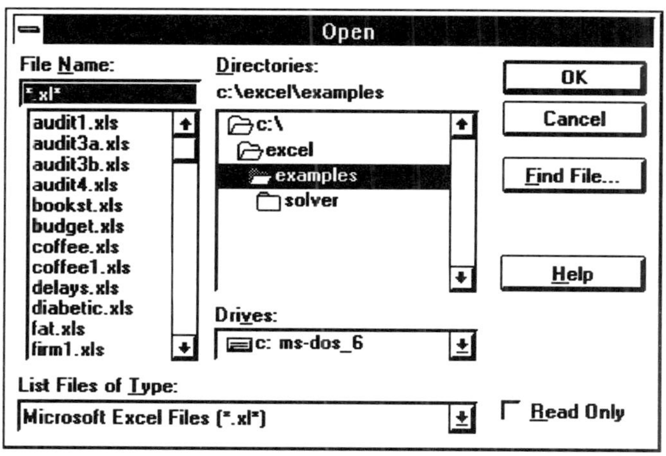

Fig. 2.2 The Open dialog box.

Hint: If you store your files in different directories, you may need to select from the directory box or drive box if the file you require is not in the current directory or drive. You may also have to slide down the scroll bar if the file you require is not currently showing in the file selection box.

There is now a spreadsheet available for use which should look like the following.

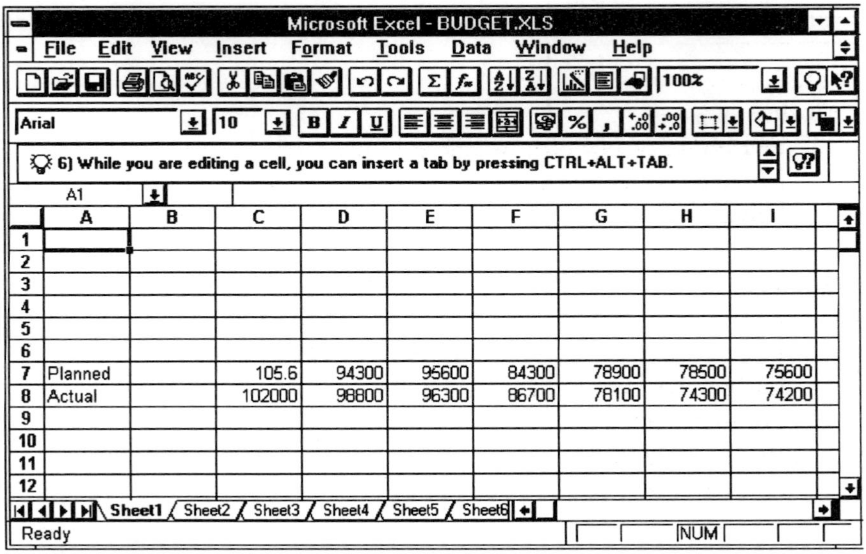

Fig. 2.3 Basic budget data in BUDGET.XLS.

2.2.2 Entering labels

First we need to enter a title for our sheet:

🖱 **Click** on B3.

☛ **Type** Planned & Actual Expenditure, Newtown Practice, 1994.

☛ **Press** ↵.

Do not be concerned about the title flooding over into adjacent cells.

2.2.3 Entering Data

The figures for the first month in column B are omitted. We shall enter them now:

🖱 **Click** on B7.

☛ **Type** 98800↵.

> **Hint**: Pressing ↵ will enter the data in a cell and move down a row.

☛ **Type** 100300↵ .

Hint: If you are worried about typing errors then mistakes are easily corrected:

Double-click on cell containing incorrect text (B3 in this case)
Move the I-bar pointer to the immediate right of the error.
Click (note that another flashing bar I appears within the text)

The flashing bar can be moved using keyboard arrow keys if incorrectly placed.

Use ← and [Del] keys to remove characters to the left or right of flashing bar respectively.
To insert characters just type them in.
Press ↵ to end edit or **press** [Esc] to end edit and retain the original text.

Alternatively, to use the method retained from older versions of Excel (and the only method available to users of Excel 4.0 or earlier), then

Click on B3
Move the I-bar pointer to the editing bar immediately above the sheet where the text is displayed.
Move the I-bar pointer to the immediate right of the error.
Click (note that another flashing bar I appears within the text).
The flashing bar can be moved using keyboard arrow keys if incorrectly placed.
Use ← and [Del] keys to remove characters to the left or right of flashing bar respectively.
To insert characters just type them in.
Click on ☑ or **Press** ↵ to end edit, or
Click on ☒ or **Press** [Esc] to end edit and retain the original text.

2.2.4 Formulae

Now we shall enter our first formula. This is important, because this is where the computer starts to do the work. The art of using a spreadsheet is constructive laziness: never do yourself what the computer could do for you!

First of all we shall calculate the size of the over- or under-spend for each month. In column A we will add a label:

🖱 **Click** on A10.

☛ **Type** Budget Variance.

☛ **Press** ⇥ .

You should now be at cell B10.

> **Hint:** Remember ↵ enters text and moves down a cell; ⇥ enters text and moves to the right.

To calculate the under/over budget figure:

☛ **Type** =.

This tells Excel that this is a formula, not a number or label. Excel places the Function Wizard button at the beginning of the edit line.

🖱 **Click** on B7.

The cell becomes outlined and the cell reference is entered in B10:

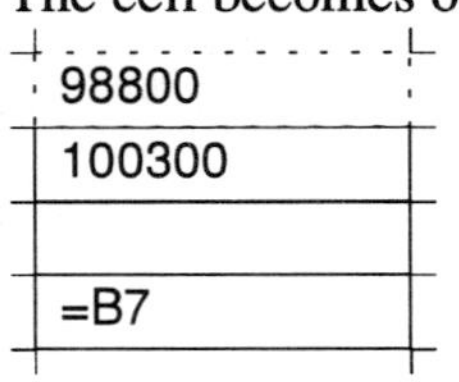

Fig. 2.4 Entering the formula in cell B10.

☛ **Type** -. (a minus sign)

🖱 **Click** on B8.

☛ **Press** ↵.

The formula in cell B10 should now have changed to a number as the computer calculates the answer straight away. The answer should be -1500. Note that the value appears in the cell, but the formula remains displayed on the edit line. Any future change to the values of the cells will cause the cell to be re-calculated automatically. To enter a formula this way for a lot of numbers would be tedious but we can 'copy' formulae across a row or down a column.

Click on B10.

Note that in the bottom right-hand corner of the highlighted cell there is a little black square which changes to a small black cross as the cursor moves over it:

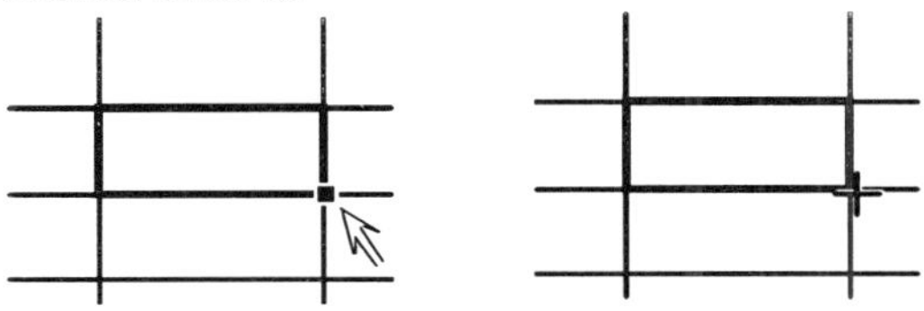

Fig. 2.5 Engaging the Autofill function

If the cross is dragged to the right we can outline a row from B10 to M10.

-1500											

When the mouse button is released then the sheet automatically fills the cells outlined.

-1500	3600	-4500	-700	-2400	800	4200	1400	2000	-2100	1200	3200

Move the pointer away and **click** on another cell to remove the highlighting.

This is Excel's Autofill function which is easy to use and of which more will be heard later.

Health Warning:	Autofill is not always appropriate for your calculations. Check them carefully by looking at the formulae on the edit line.

Two alternative methods can be used. These should be used when Autofill is not appropriate. The first is as follows:

Click on B10.

Click on (copy) from the toolbar.

Note that an outline marquee appears around B10.

Paint C10 to M10.

Click on (paste) from the toolbar.

Press [Esc] to remove the outline marquee around B10.

As always, there is an alternative to the toolbar within the menus

Click on B10.

Select 'Edit' from the menu bar.

Select 'Copy'.

Paint C10 to M10.

Select 'Edit' from the menu bar.

Select 'Paste'.

Press [Esc] to remove the outline marquee around B10.

The formula will now have been copied to the appropriate cells.

Health Warning: Check the formulae to make sure that they are correct.

If we wish to calculate the over- or under-budget as a percentage of the whole budget, then we may do this in row 12:

Click on A12.

Type Over/Under % variance .

Click on B12.

Type = .

Click on B10.

Type / .

Click on B7 ↵.

Hint: As a formula is copied across it changes. For example, if a formula in B2 is =B1*6 then if we copy it across a row it will become =C1*6 in C2, =D1*6 in D2 and so on.

2		=B1*6	=C1*6	=D1*6	=E1*6

Similarly, if we copy the formula down, it will change. If a formula in B2 reads =A2/6, then in B3, the formula will read =A3/6 and so on.

2		=A2/6
3		=A3/6
4		=A4/6
5		=A5/6
6		=A6/6

This is an example of relative references. To fix a reference to a cell so that it does not change we prefix it by a dollar sign. Thus if we copy the formula '=$A$2+42' across or down it will always read '=$A$2+42'.

2		=$A$2+42	=$A$2+42	=$A$2+42	=$A$2+42
3		=$A$2+42			
4		=$A$2+42			
5		=$A$2+42			
6		=$A$2+42			

We shall use absolute references later, starting in Chapter 4.

This produces figures which have excessive accuracy. This problem will be dealt with later in this chapter. We can also change this decimal fraction to a percentage.

We can now copy this formula by using Autofill (or one of the alternatives) as above. Try this as your first exercise on your own. The final results should look like this:

-0.01518	0.034091	-0.04772	-0.00732	-0.02847	0.010139	0.053503	*etc.*

As always, check the formulae (in the edit bar above the sheet) to make sure that they are correct.

Autofill can also be used to provide the headings for our sheet:

🖱 **Click** on B5.

☛ **Type** Jan↵.

🖱 **Click** on B5.

🖱 **Autofill** from B5 across to M5.

> **Hint:** From now on in the text, we shall simply refer to the Autofill operation as a single instruction: remember it means dragging the little black square from the bottom right corner of the cell. See above if you are not sure.

The row should now have the month labels through to December in cells B5 to M5. Excel enters the monthly headings because it recognizes ‘Jan’ as the first of a sequence. It will also recognize the full names of days and months and the first three letters of any day or month.

For completeness,

🖱 **Click** on N5.

☛ **Type** Total↵.

2.2.5 Moving Around the Spreadsheet

> **Hint:** To return to the top left hand corner of the sheet at any time:
> ☛ **Press** [Ctrl] and [Home] together.

We have already seen that it is easy to move around the spreadsheet using the scroll bars. In a large sheet it can be quite tedious to do this if you know that you want to alter information in one particular cell. To move to a specific cell, e.g. B3:

Click on 'Edit' from the menu bar.

Click on 'Go to'.

or alternatively,

Press [F5].

Either should bring the 'Go to' dialog box onto the screen.

Type B3↵.

Click on [OK].

2.3 EVALUATING THE YEAR'S PERFORMANCE

Spreadsheets contain a number of functions, essentially pre-programmed formulae, thus saving the user time in thinking and typing out the formulae in detail.

Press [F5].

Type N7↵.

Click on [Σ] on the toolbar.

Press ↵ to confirm the formula suggested.

This function may be used to total any row or column of figures. In Excel 4 it could only be used on individual cells, but now it can be used to sum sets of rows or columns. If you sum a set of rows, Excel will not prompt you for confirmation of the formulae. Thus, to illustrate this:

Click on N7.

Press [Del].

Paint cells N7 and N8.

Click on [Σ] on the toolbar.

The answer appears without prompting:

Health Warning: Autosum (Σ)cannot be used where the cells are non-adjacent.

As always there is an alternative via the menus, in this case the 'Insert' menu, shown in Fig. 2.6. (Note that this is one place where Excel 5.0 differs radically from earlier versions.)

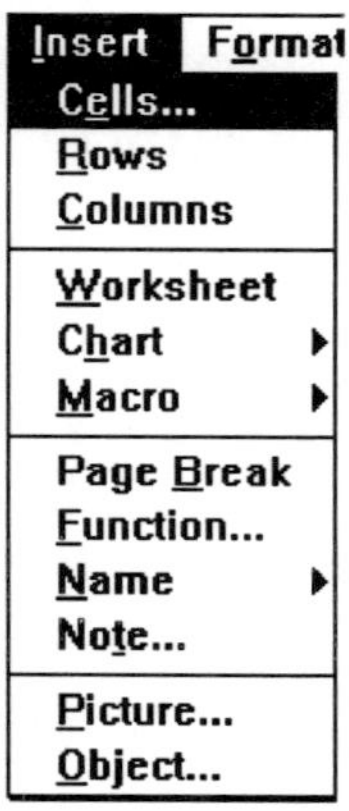

Fig. 2.6 The Insert menu.

Remove the existing formulae:

☛ **Press** [Del].

Identify the cell where the formula is to go:

🖱 **Click** on N7.

🖱 **Select** 'Insert' from the menu bar.

🖱 **Select** 'Function' from the menu bar.

This produces the Function Wizard dialog box, shown in Fig. 2.7. Wizards are part of Excel and they are designed to guide us through the process of constructing a formula.

Hint: A shortcut way to the Function Wizard is through the Function Wizard toolbar button [fx].

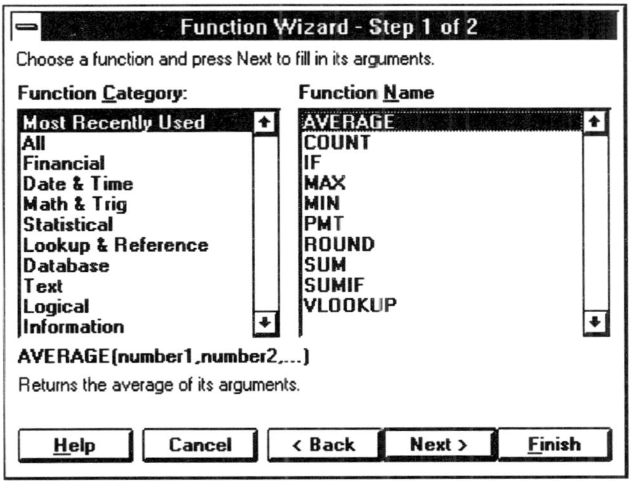

Fig. 2.7 The function Wizard dialog box

The system organizes the available functions into categories and displays the most recently used. As 'Sum' appears in this list:

- **Select** 'Sum'.
- **Click** on Next >.

  Now enter the range required:

- **Type** B7:M7 ↵.

then to finish the process:.

- **Click** on Finish.

This formula can be copied to cells N8 and N10 simultaneously:

- **Click** on N7.
- **Click** on  from the toolbar.
- **Click** on N8 .
- **Hold down** [Ctrl].
- **Click** on N10.
- **Click** on 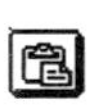 from the toolbar.
- **Press** [Esc] to remove the outline marquee.

As always, there is an alternative to the toolbar within the menus

- **Click** on N7.
- **Select** 'Edit' from the menu bar.
- **Select** 'Copy'.
- **Click** on N8 .
- **Hold down** [Ctrl].
- **Click** on N10.
- **Select** 'Edit' from the menu bar.
- **Select** 'Paste'.
- **Press** [Esc] to remove the outline marquee.

To complete the sheet, copy the formula in M12 to N12.

2.4 IMPROVING PRESENTATION

2.4.1 To change column widths

The first column containing the labels is too narrow. We can change its width by using the mouse:

- **Move** the cursor to column label A at the top of the first column.
- **Move** to right-hand side of cell between column A and column B:

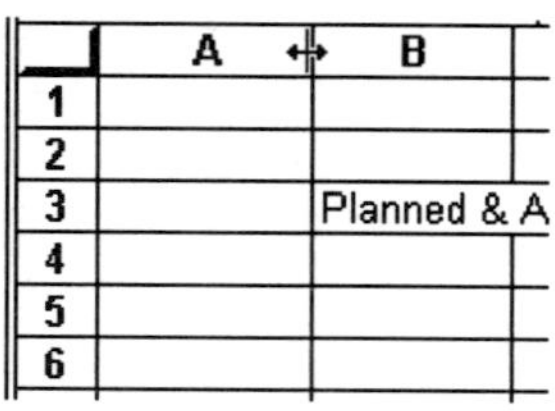

Fig. 2.8 Changing the column width via the mouse.

Note that the 'cross' pointer changes to an 'iron cross'.

- **Drag** the iron cross cursor to the right.

A faint vertical grey line appears below the cross as the mouse moves to the right. The column will widen when you release the button.

A second way to change the column width is to place the cursor as above, but to double-click instead of dragging. This will perform a 'best fit' to accommodate the entries in the column.

Double-click on the line between columns A and B in the header row.

Health Warning:	Sometimes 'best fit' can have unexpected results: try widening column B using this method to see what happens!

As usual, there is a further range of options available from the menus. To find them:

Select 'Format' from the menu bar.

Select 'Column'.

Select 'Width'.

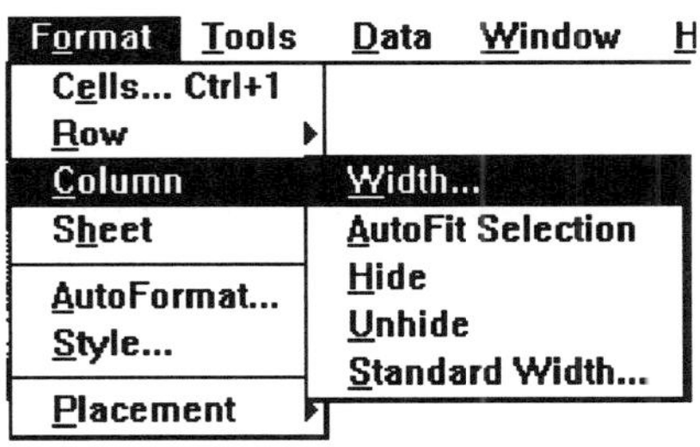

Fig. 2.9 The column option on the Format menu.

Type 6.

Click on OK.

2.4.2 Formatting text

We can change many other aspects of presentation either from the tool bars or from a short cut menu or from the Format menu. Most of the formatting option toolbar buttons appear on the Ribbon below the main toolbar shown in Fig. 2.10.

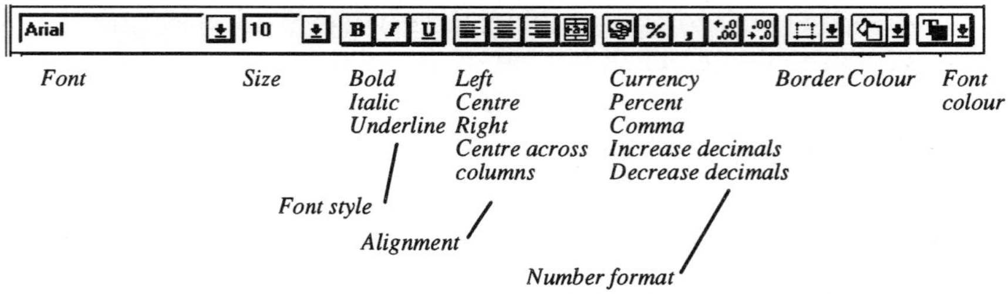

Fig. 2.10 Format options on the ribbon below the main toolbar.

One of the simplest formatting operations is the alignment of text. Text may be left- right- or centre- aligned. To illustrate this, highlight the month labels in our budget sheet:

- **Paint** B5 to N5.
- **Click** on .

The titles are now right-aligned with the numbers below.

With the cells still highlighted,

- **Click** on  to centre-align the cells and then
- **Click** on  to left-align the cells.

An alternative approach is to access the Format Cells dialog box, shown in Fig. 2.11. The easiest way is:

With the cells still highlighted:

- **Select** 'Format' from the menu bar.
- **Select** 'Cells'.
- **Select** Alignment.
- **Select** 'Right' from the horizontal options.
- **Click** on OK.

We can select left or centre alignment in a similar fashion. Try it now for practice.

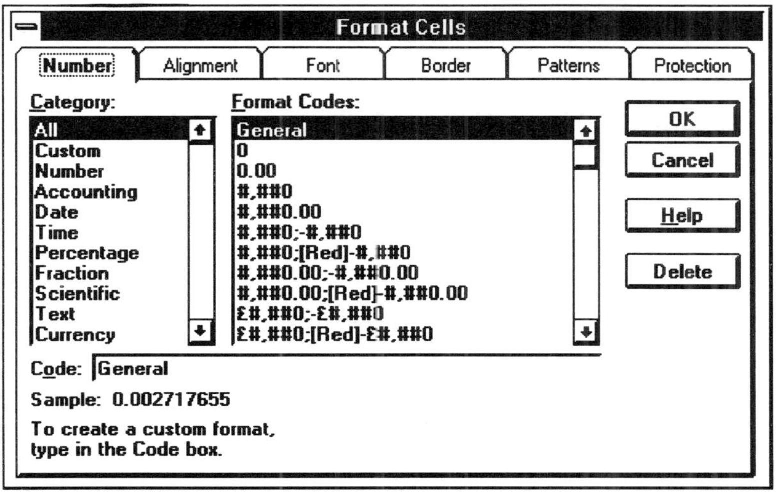

Fig. 2.11 The Format Cells dialog box.

The other major formatting option available for text is the style of text. To change our month headings to italics, highlight the range B5 to M5 if not already highlighted, then

Click on *I*.

If we repeat the action, the italics are removed:

Click on *I*.

To embolden the text,

Click on **B**.

Now if we italicize the text, we get both bold and italics:

Click on *I*.

The titles should now look like:

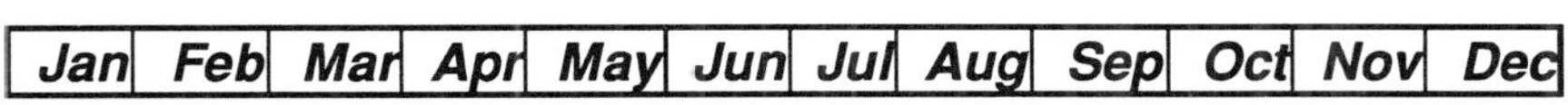

Hint: The same result can be achieved from the keyboard. With the cells still highlighted:

Press [Ctrl] and B together.

Press [Ctrl] and I together.

We can change the font size using the drop down box containing the point size located near to the font display:

Click on ⯆ next to the point size box.

Select '12' from the drop down list.

> **Hint**: There is a keyboard shortcut for this, which may be quicker:
>
> ☛ **Press** [Ctrl] and [Shift] and P together
>
> ☛ **Type** 12↵

> **Health Warning**: Keyboard shortcuts are fast if you can remember them, but can be confusing if not. Using the mouse is often easier for inexperienced users.

The font may also be changed from the drop down list. The current font name is 'Arial'. To change the titles to Times New Roman. With the cells still highlighted:

Click on ⯆ next to the font name box.

Select 'Times New Roman' from the drop down list.

All these options and more may accessed from the Font tab in the Format cells dialog box. To examine these options:

With the cells still highlighted:.

Select 'Format' from the menu bar.

Select 'Cells'.

Select [Font].

As an exercise, see if you can restore the headings to Arial 10pt Bold using the dialog box.

2.4.3 Formatting numbers

It is useful in financial statements to use standard accounting formats: to insert Pound signs, to add commas after thousands and millions. If we wish to be really smart, we may show losses in parentheses or (if we have a colour screen) in red. The first stage is most easily accomplished by using the toolbar.

☛ **Paint** B7 to N10.

Click on .

Initially the results do not appear too promising, producing a series of cells containing #########. This indicates that the entries are too wide for the columns. The currency button sets the format to pounds and pence, with commas at thousands and millions, thus 100300 becomes £100,300.00. We shall reduce this to include only pounds, using the decrease decimal button:

Click on twice.

An alternative, if we wish to retain the full format, is to widen the columns as above.

To display our deficit in red, we must go back to the Format Cells dialog box:

With the cells still highlighted:

Select 'Format' from the menu bar.

Select 'Cells'.

Select Number.

Select 'Currency'.

Select '£#, ##0; [RED] £#, ##0'.

Click on OK.

Notice that in those months where the budget is overspent, the figures now appear in red on the screen.

Health Warning: Most people print in black and white, which will not show colour effects. It may be better to show a deficit in parentheses.

Hint: The country is set up in the Windows environment. If you experience problems getting a £ sign at the keyboard or screen, then check your country settings. Look for (the Control Panel) in the Program Manager and choose to change the country settings.

The percentage variances are currently shown as decimals. We can change these to percentages and show the negatives in parentheses:

- **Paint** B12 to N12.
- **Click** on .
- **Click** on twice to show to two decimal places.

As an exercise, try to reformat the range B10 to M10 so that negatives appear in brackets as well as red using the above method.

2.4.4 Gridlines

In a final statement, it would not generally be appropriate to have gridlines displayed. They can be removed as follows:

- **Select** 'Tools' from the menu bar.
- **Select** 'Options'.

The dialog box, shown in Fig. 2.12, gives access to a vast range of customization options.

- **Select** [View].
- **Select** 'Gridlines'.
- **Click** on [OK].

Hint: The cross in the box will be removed to indicate that the 'Gridlines' option is de-selected.

2.4.5 Borders

We may still wish to highlight certain areas by use of a border:

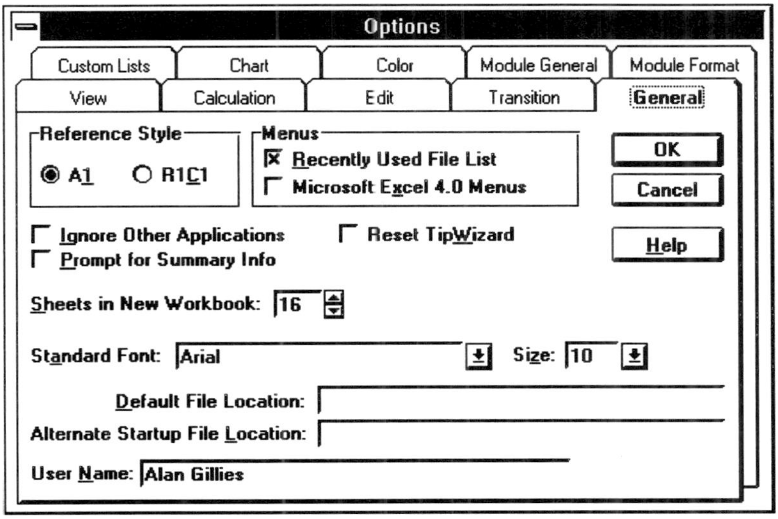

Fig. 2.12 The Options dialog box.

☛ **Paint** the area A12 to N12.

🖱 **Click** on the arrow next to the border button in the tool bar.

This produces a range of border options.

🖱 **Click** on the bottom right-hand option.

A simple border will now surround the painted area. The border button changes as the border itself changes.

Now try some of the more complex options:

🖱 **Click** on the arrow next to the border button in the tool bar.

🖱 **Click** on some of the other options displayed to see their effect.

For complete flexibility, we can select the Border tab from the Format Cells dialog box:

With the cells still highlighted:

🖱 **Select** 'Format' from the menu bar.

🖱 **Select** 'Cells'.

🖱 **Select** Border.

By painting different areas of the screen and using this option we can have almost complete control over the borders displayed.

2.4.6 Autoformatting

Excel provides a range of built-in formats for sheets to provide an easy way of improving presentation.

Paint A3 to N12.

Select 'Format' from the command bar.

Select 'Autoformat'.

A dialog box appears as shown in Fig. 2.13. Examine some of the available options.

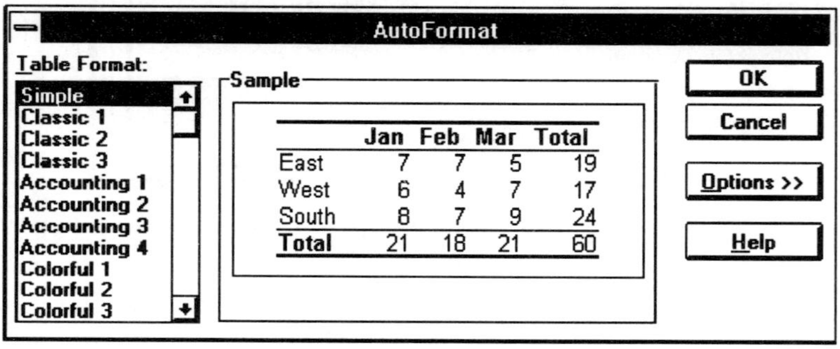

Fig. 2.13 The Autoformat dialog box.

Select 'Colourful2'.

Click on [OK].

This should have a fairly dramatic effect. However many autoformats will need tweaking to be really useful. Some of the simpler formats are actually the most effective. If the cell range is not already selected,

Paint A3 to N12.

Now apply the 'Simple' Autoformat. Check all the numerical formats, some will need changing back to their correct format.

2.5 WHEN YOU'RE HAPPY WITH IT

2.5.1 Printing the completed sheet

If we simply want to print a sheet we can use the print button on the toolbar:

Click on [print icon].

However, generally it is worth having a look at the result first on the screen. To achieve this,

Click on [print preview icon] (print preview) which is next to the Print button on the toolbar.

This allows us to preview what the printed version will look like. Note that the pointer changes to a magnifying glass.

Select 'Setup' and we can change almost anything about the way the sheet is printed.

The setup option is accessed by a dialog box with four tabs:

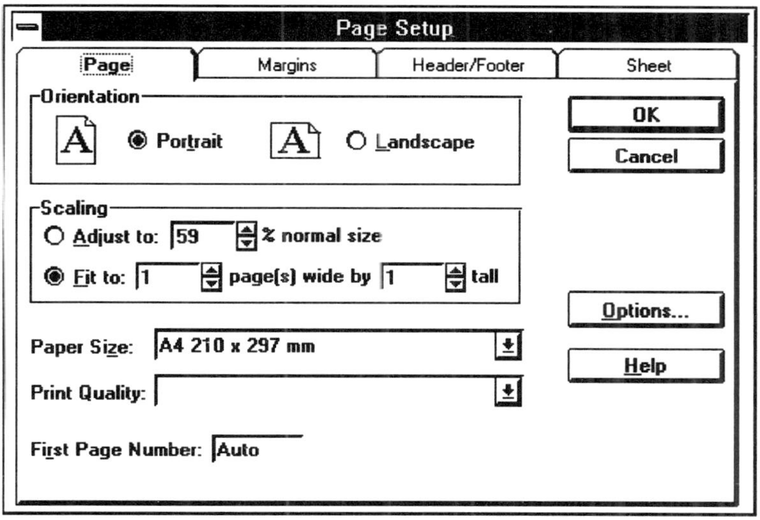

Fig. 2.14 Page Setup dialog box.

One of the most useful options is the scaling option which allows us either to specify a scaling factor or to fit the sheet automatically to a number of pages. Note that all changes are shown on the preview screen.

The printed dialog box shows the 'Fit to'option set up to scale our budget sheet to fit on one page.

To achieve this,

Click in the circle next to 'Fit to'.

Click on [OK] to accept the default of 1 page wide by 1 page tall.

Another feature which is useful is the Margins option.

Click on Margins.

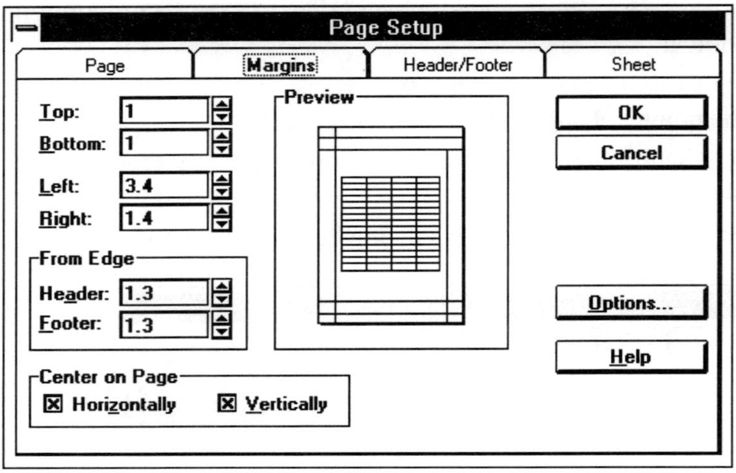

Fig. 2.15 Dialog box accessed from the Margins tab.

This allows us to see the exact margins at the sides, top and bottom of each printed sheet. This is particularly useful if the size of the printed worksheet needs to be expanded. By dragging on the small square boxes the margin can be moved about the page.

Click on Header/Footer.

These options, accessed via the dialog box shown in Fig. 2.16, control the header and footer that are printed with the sheet. You may include the date, the page number, the file name and any text.

Once the setup options are set, then the worksheet may be printed from within the main preview dialog box:

Click on Print.

The Print dialog box appears, as shown in Fig. 2.17.

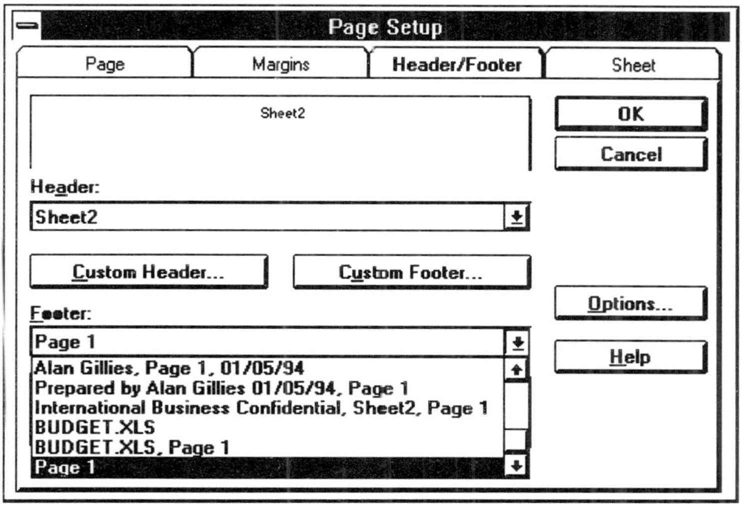

Fig. 2.16 Dialog box accessed from the Header/Footer tab.

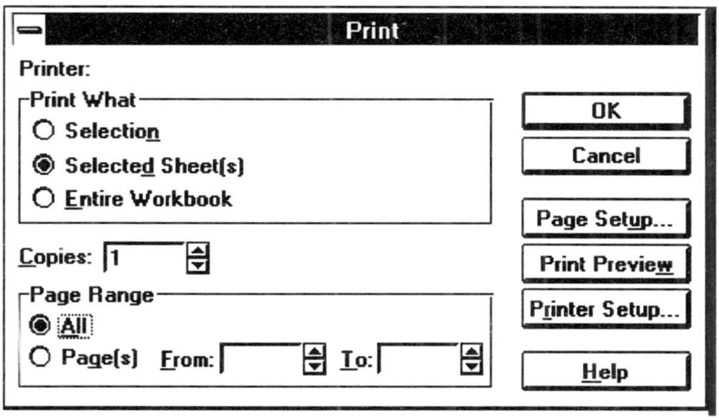

Fig. 2.17 The Print dialog box.

Hint: The name of the printer in use will appear at the top of the box next to the word printer, e.g. Hewlett Packard LJIII+ on LPT1:

At this stage, we have options to print, a selection, a sheet or the entire collection of sheets known as a workbook. Within this, we have the option to print all the pages or a selected range. The buttons on the right allow us to access the preview facility, or to change the page or printer setup.

Health Warning: Printing in Excel is controlled by the Windows Print Manager. If you experience problems with printing then check that your printer matches that specified by the system. To do this:

- **Click** on 'Print'
- **Click** on 'Printer Setup'

If you need to set up a new printer and it is not already listed you may need the original Windows disks to copy over a new printer driver.

If the printer is set up correctly and the page is set up according to our wishes, then all we need to do is to

- **Click** on [OK] to print our sheet.

2.5.2 Saving the Sheet

Before we leave Excel, we must save our work to the hard disk inside the computer, so that we may retrieve it at a later date. Because we wish to save the work under a different name from the original sheet, we must use the 'Save as'option under the File menu:

- **Select** 'File' from the menu bar.
- **Select** 'Save As'.
- **Type** budget1.xls↵.

The worksheet is now saved in a file in the Excel directory called 'budget1.xls'.

Hint: When you leave Excel, if you have not saved any changes, the system will prompt you to make changes. This is another 'have you lost your presence of mind?' message. Ignore it at your peril!

If we wish to save it in future, to the same filename, all we have to do is:

- **Click** on [save icon] on the toolbar.

Excel also allows us to save our data in other formats to allow transfer of data to other packages, such as Lotus 1-2-3, Dbase II, III or

IV, as well as previous versions of Excel. For example, to save our data as a Lotus worksheet which may be read by a wide range of other packages, as well as Lotus 1-2-3, first ensure that the data sheet is on top:

Select 'File' from the menu bar.

Select 'Save As'.

Type budget1.wks.

Select WKS(1-2-3) from the drop down list of file types.

The completed dialog box should now look like Fig. 2.18:

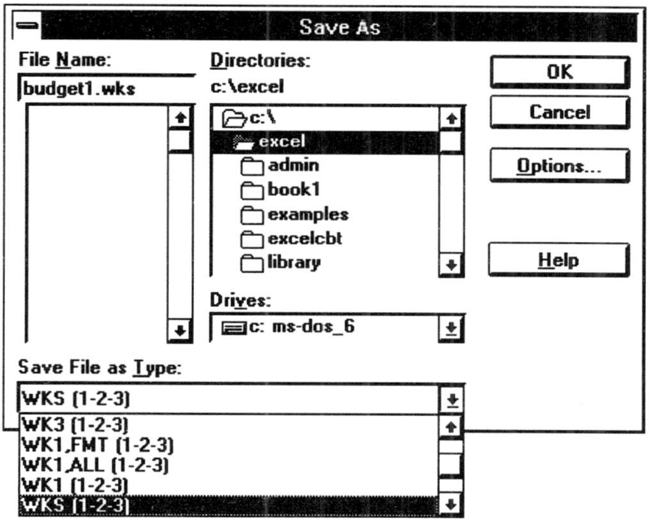

Fig. 2.18 The Save As dialog box.

Click on [OK].

Health Warning: Saving data in other formats is subject to some limitations, notably many foreign formats only save one sheet. Further, some formatting information such as fonts may be lost.

3

Presenting the budget results to colleagues

3.1 CHAPTER SUMMARY

Having set up a sheet to monitor discrepancies between planned and actual expenditure, it may be necessary to produce results for colleagues. The simplest way to display such findings is in graphical format. In this chapter we shall demonstrate how to use Excel to

- display the budget data in graphical format; and how to
- choose an appropriate graph.

In the process we shall introduce the following features of Excel:

- producing 2-dimensional graphs in Excel;
- producing 3-dimensional graphs in Excel;
- graph formatting;
- displaying graphs within spreadsheets.

3.2 PRESENTING DATA WITH EXCEL

Excel has excellent graphing procedures which require very little effort to use if you know what you are doing! There are a wide variety of different graphs available for use according to the nature of the data which we wish to represent, all of which can be presented in two and three dimensions.

3.2.1 Bar / line charts

This type of chart may be used to show a data set over a period of time (a year in months, 5 years in yearly intervals or in quarters). Generally bars may be used for 1, 2 or 3 data sets but become unmanageable for 4 or more data sets. Bars are useful for month-by-month comparisons of two or three data sets. Line charts which represent the data as a set of points, can be more useful than bars when looking at a trend over time.

3.2.2 Pie charts

This type of graph is useful for showing proportions or distributions. For example we may depict how FHSA fees and allowances are distributed between categories such as capitation fees, basic practice allowances, immunizations and vaccinations, etc.

3.2.3 Area charts

This type of chart is useful when it is used to highlight not only the data series but also the area underneath the points and can show the difference between two series.

3.2.4 X–Y Charts

X–Y charts allow us to examine the relationship between an independent and a dependent variable. Such visual inspection is useful before conducting correlation or regression analysis and may reveal whether further statistical analysis is worth pursuing.

3.3 COMPARING PLANNED AND ACTUAL EXPENDITURE

To help develop an understanding of how charts and graphs may be used to illustrate practice reports, the following examples will be used to demonstrate how the simple budgets shown in the previous chapter may be enhanced. The first example to be used is that of Planned and Actual Expenditure shown in the previous chapter and to be found under the saved filename of budget1.xls. If your sheet is incomplete, you may use budget2.xls which is a completed version supplied on the disk:

- **Click** on [Open button].
- **Select** either budget1.xls or budget2.xls as appropriate.
- **Click** on [OK].

As already indicated, a line graph is an appropriate method of illustrating differences in planned and actual expenditure for a practice. To produce the graph we shall use the ChartWizard in Excel which produces a chart embedded in the worksheet.

The ChartWizard is, to quote Microsoft:

' a set of dialog boxes that simplifies creating a chart'.

We can create our chart within the existing sheet or as a separate sheet. We shall first create a chart in the same sheet as the data. Before we draw the chart, we need to highlight the appropriate data. In this case we wish to look at the picture for the whole year but to help clarify the graph we should also like to include the 'month' labels and use the row labels as legends. The relevance will be seen later.

- **Paint** A5 to M5 .
- **Hold down** the [Ctrl] key and
- **Paint** A7 to M8.
- **Click** on [ChartWizard button].

This is the ChartWizard Button, and it is found towards the right side of the standard toolbar.

> **Health warning**: This can be tricky. With the [Ctrl] key held down it is easy to paint the wrong cells as you move back to the left. It is therefore recommended that you move the mouse pointer back to column A before you hold down the [Ctrl] key and the left mouse key.

The 'arrow' icon changes to a graph icon: .

Choose a point on the screen towards top left then

- **Hold down** the left mouse button.
- **Drag** the graph icon towards bottom left to create a chart box and release the mouse button when a suitable size of box is created. .

The ChartWizard guides you through five steps to produce a graph:

- Step 1: Choose data range (if necessary), **Click** on [Next >].
- Step 2: Choose graph type, **Click** on [Next >].
- Step 3: Choose graph format, **Click** on [Next >].
- Step 4: Data series format (rows or columns), **Click** on [Next >].
- Step 5: Add legend, **Click** on [Finish].

The complete ChartWizard cycle is shown in Fig. 3.1.

The graph will now appear complete with the 'month' labels along the horizontal axis. Embedding the chart in the same sheet as the data is convenient for viewing, but we can do more if we place it on a separate sheet. For convenience, delete the embedded chart by

- **Press** [Del] with the chart selected.
- **Paint** A5 to M5 .
- **Hold down** the [Ctrl] key and **paint** A7 to M8.
- **Select** 'Insert' from the menu bar.
- **Select** 'Chart'.
- **Select** 'As New Sheet'.

> **Hint:** To shortcut this process, paint your data sheet and then press [F11] to replace the last three instructions.

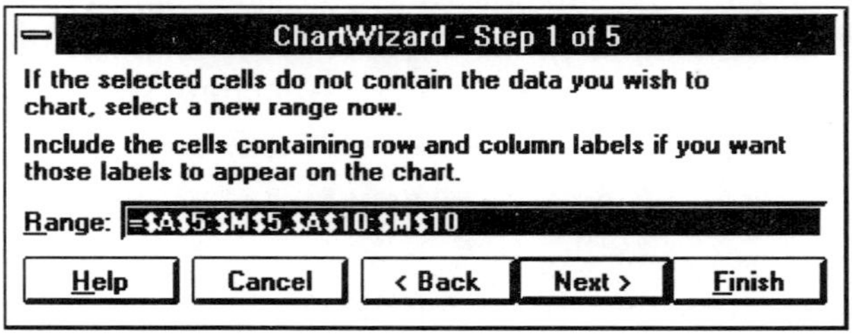
ChartWizard - Step 1 of 5
If the selected cells do not contain the data you wish to chart, select a new range now.
Include the cells containing row and column labels if you want those labels to appear on the chart.
Range: =$A$5:$M$5,$A$10:$M$10
Help
Cancel
< Back
Next >
Finish

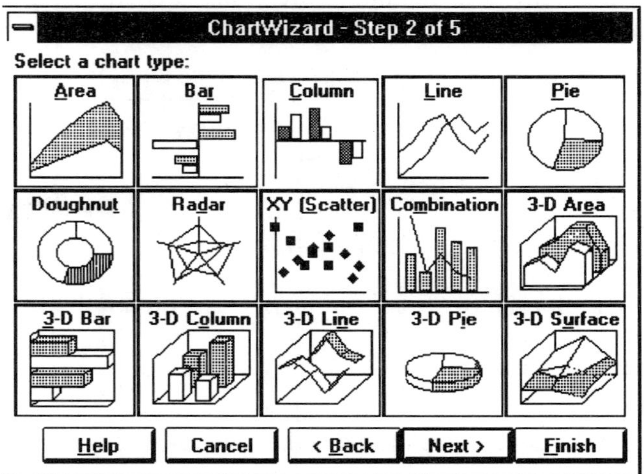
ChartWizard - Step 2 of 5
Select a chart type:
Area
Bar
Column
Line
Pie
Doughnut
Radar
XY (Scatter)
Combination
3-D Area
3-D Bar
3-D Column
3-D Line
3-D Pie
3-D Surface
Help
Cancel
< Back
Next >
Finish

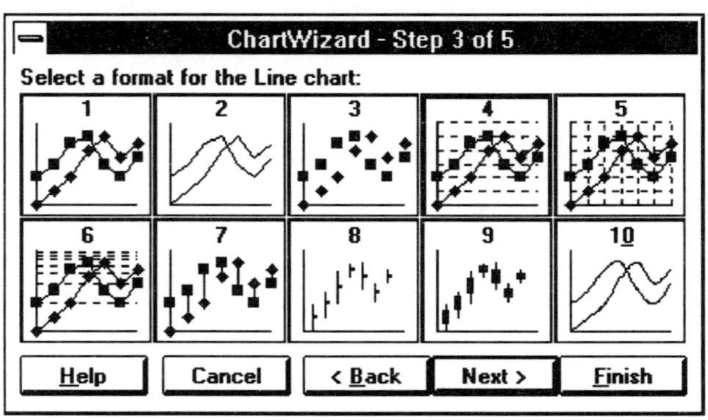
ChartWizard - Step 3 of 5
Select a format for the Line chart:
1
2
3
4
5
6
7
8
9
10
Help
Cancel
< Back
Next >
Finish

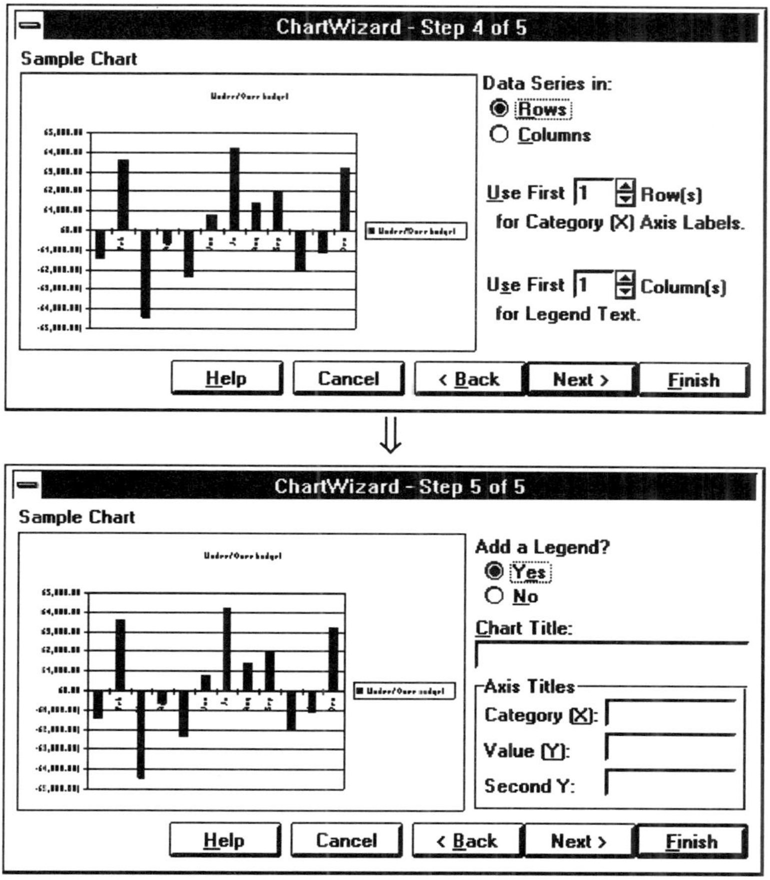

Fig. 3.1 The five stages of ChartWizard.

Now we could repeat steps 1 to 5 through the ChartWizard, but we can save ourselves some work by selecting Finish at step 1:

Click on [Finish].

The same chart as before is now found on a separate sheet, named Chart1.

If we wish to produce any more charts from this worksheet, the ChartWizard will use the format that we have now established. We shall demonstrate this later when we plot the budget variance figures.

To display the data sheet,

Click on [Sheet1] at the bottom of the sheet.

To then return to the chart,

Click on Chart1 at the bottom of the sheet.

The chart may now be altered in a wide variety of ways. These items are all selected by identifying the element of the graph to be altered and then using the menus or the charting toolbar to alter that feature. In the following we shall demonstrate a range of improvements and changes which can be made:

- changing the graph type;
- using the toolbar to select a range of charts;
- adding and removing the labels and legends;
- adding text to the chart;
- adding an arrow to highlight key information.

3.4 IMPROVING THE GRAPHICAL REPRESENTATION

There are many ways in which graphical representation can be enhanced to improve the way data can be depicted. With all such improvements care has to be exercised that the enhancement is not in fact confusing the issue. Too many enhancements can make the graph look 'busy' and detract from the message being conveyed.

As usual, Excel offers us a variety of routes to achieve these results:

- main menus;
- chart toolbar;
- keyboard commands;
- shortcut menus.

In this case, the easiest route is often by the shortcut menus obtained by using the right-hand mouse button.

3.4.1 Graph type

Using the ChartWizard has resulted in Excel defaulting to a bar chart but a line graph may be more appropriate:

Right-click on the chart background.

You can tell if you have achieved the right result because the chart is outlined and the shortcut menu that appears is shown in Fig 3.2.

If you right-click on a bar or axis, then this element of the chart will be highlighted and a different shortcut menu will appear.

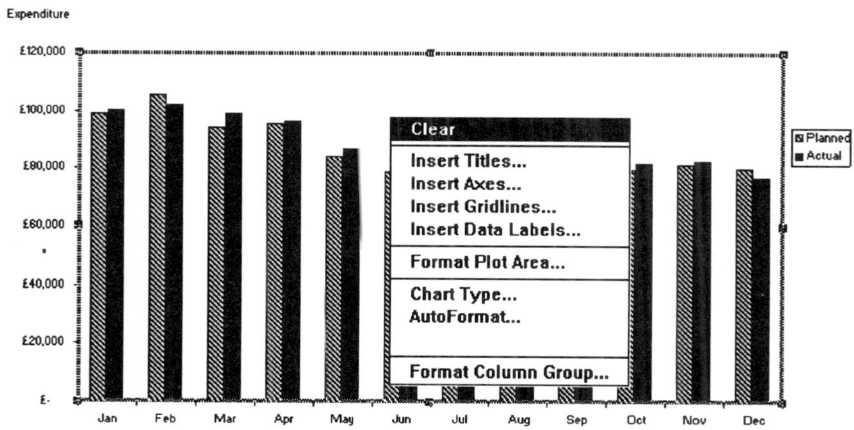

Fig. 3.2 Chart with whole chart selected and short cut menu

Select Chart type.

The dialog box that appears is shown in Fig 3.3

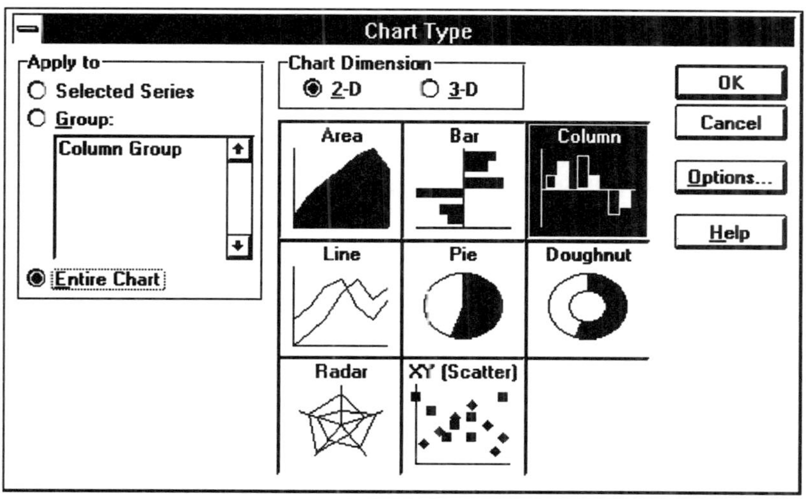

Fig. 3.3 The Chart Type dialog box.

Double-click on 'Line'.

> **Hint:** This is a quicker way of selecting the chart type and avoids the need to **click** on OK. It is equivalent to
>
> **Select** 'Line'.
>
> **Click** on OK.

The graph changes to a line graph, as shown in Fig.3.4.

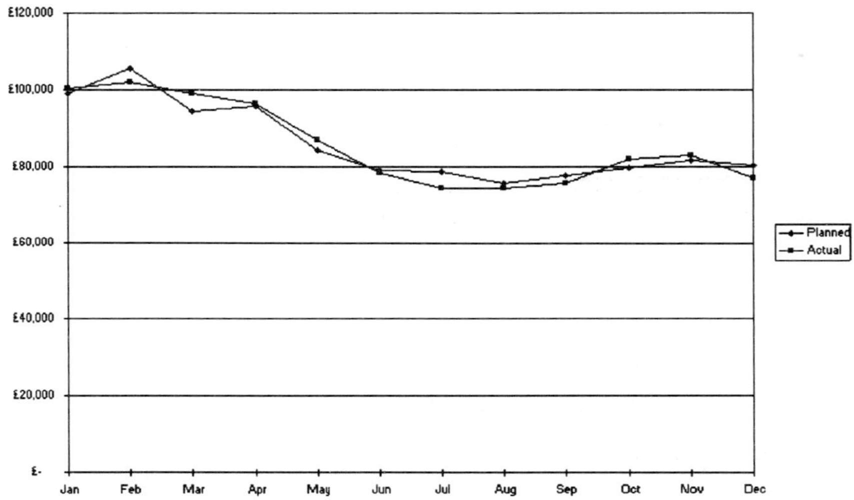

Fig. 3.4 Data displayed as a line chart.

> **Hint**: This graph illustrates the fact that it is often worth tweaking the axes' range. In this example, the Y-axis would be better restricted to £60,000 to £120,000.

You may change the format of the line chart by:

Right-click on the chart background.

Select 'Format Line Group'.

This brings up a dialog box shown in Fig. 3.5.

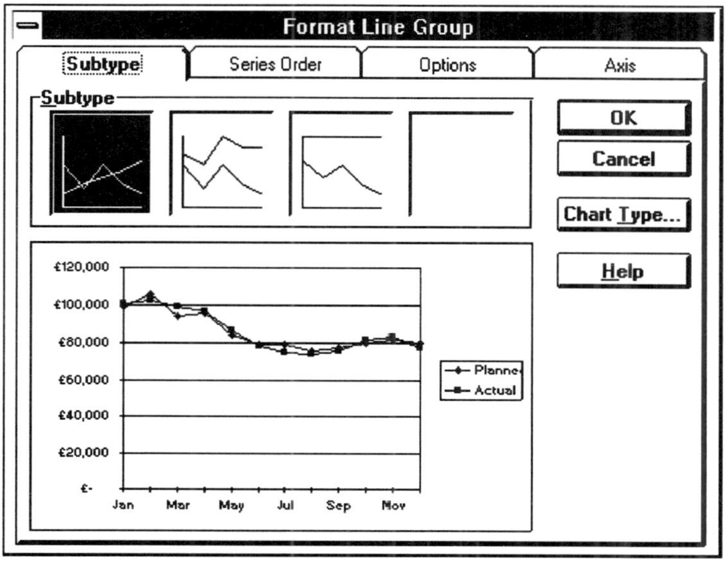

Fig. 3.5 The Format Line Group dialog box.

The subtype tab provides different types of line charts. The Series order allows you to change the order in which the data series are displayed. The options and axis features are not particularly helpful at this stage.

To change our chart back to a column chart,

- **Click** on 'Chart Type'.
- **Double-click** on 'Column'.

3.4.2 Legends

By default, the ChartWizard adds a legend to the graph at Step 5. The legend can be omitted by selecting this option at this stage. To clear the legend:

- **Click** anywhere on the legend itself. A set of black squares will surround the legend and
- **Press** [Del].

To put the legend back.

- **Select** 'Insert' from the menu bar.
- **Click** on 'Legend'.

Excel uses a default position for the legend but the position may be changed.

Click anywhere on the legend itself, if the legend is not already highlighted by a set of black squares will around it.

Drag the legend to any appropriate point on the chart.

To change the appearance of the legend,

Right-click on the legend itself.

> **Hint**: The 'Clear' option on the shortcut menu will delete the legend.

Select 'Format Legend'.

A dialog box appears with three tabs: Patterns, Font, Placement. Patterns allows you to control the border of the legend box and the area contained within it. The Font tab gives you complete control over the font used. Placement allows you to select from Bottom, Corner, Top, Left, Right. Remember that you can also place the legend anywhere on the chart by dragging it. The best way to familiarize yourself with the different options is to try different combinations.

> **Hint**: If you want to escape from a dialog box without making any changes, press [Esc].

3.4.3 Graph labelling

It is important that graphs are correctly labelled in order to state clearly the relevance of the graph.

Right-click on the chart background.

Select 'Insert Titles'.

Select 'Chart Title' by clicking on the box.

Click on OK.

The word 'Title' appears surrounded by selection panes.
Type Planned and Actual Expenditure↵

> **Hint**: The text appears in the edit bar.

To add a vertical axis title:

Right-click on the chart background.

Select 'Insert Titles'.

Select the Value (Y) Axis.

Click on OK.

Type Expenditure↵.

To add a horizontal axis title:

Right-click on the chart background.

Select 'Insert Titles'.

Select the Category (X) Axis.

Click on OK.

Type 1993↵.

Changes may be made to any one label or indeed all labels by appropriate highlighting and menu item selection. For example, should you wish to change the font size of the title:

Right-click on the chart title.

Select 'Format Chart Title'.

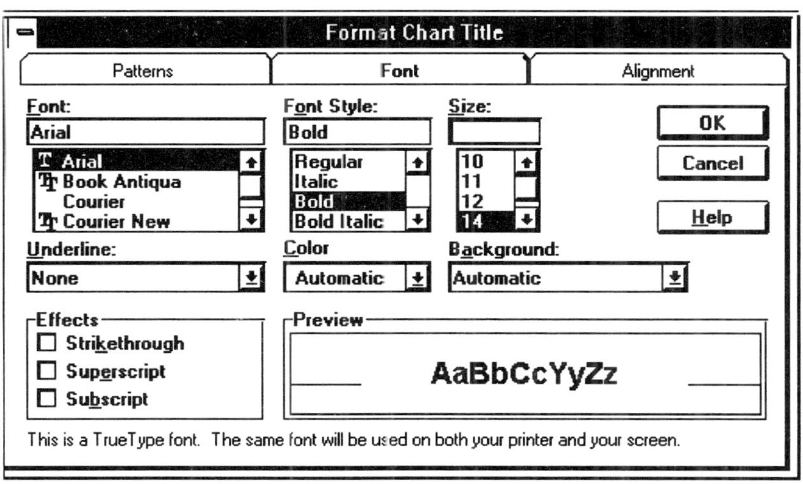

Fig. 3.6 Format Chart Title dialog box.

Select Font.

Select '14' from the Size drop down list.

Click on OK.

Alternatively, to move the Y-axis label to the top of the axis, remove the emboldening and change the text alignment to horizontal, try the following:

Right-click on the Y-axis label (Expenditure).

Select 'Format Axis Title'.

Select Font.

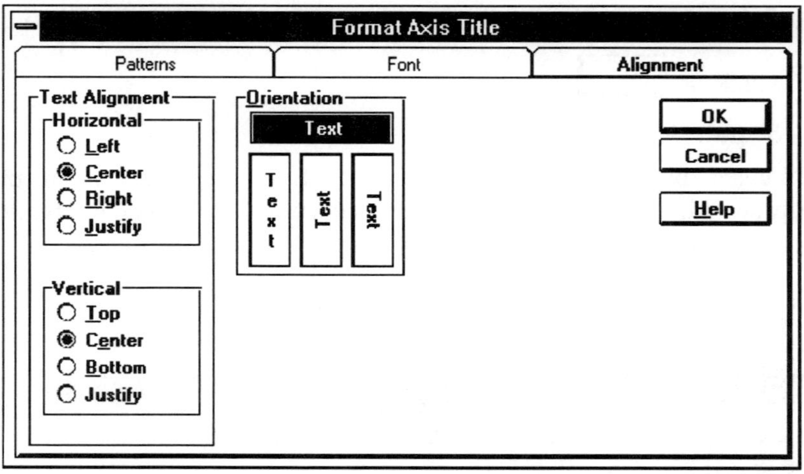

Fig. 3.7 Format axis title.

Select 'Regular' from the Font Style list.

Select Alignment.

Select 'Text' to show the text horizontally.

Click on OK.

Drag the modified label to the top of the Y-axis.

Hint: It is possible that the Y-axis title floods over into the vertical axis values. It can be dragged to a more appropriate position.

3.4.4 Colour and Hatching

Colours are useful to indicate differences between data series; in a report it is likely that all data must be shown in monochrome. In this case it is necessary to use hatch marks, to distinguish between the data series.

For example to render the current column chart suitable for monochrome printing, it is necessary to change the blue columns to a hatched pattern.

Health warning: Excessive use of colour can destroy the clarity of a graph, particularly when we come on to three dimensional charts later. Remember, the primary purpose of a graph is to COMMUNICATE!

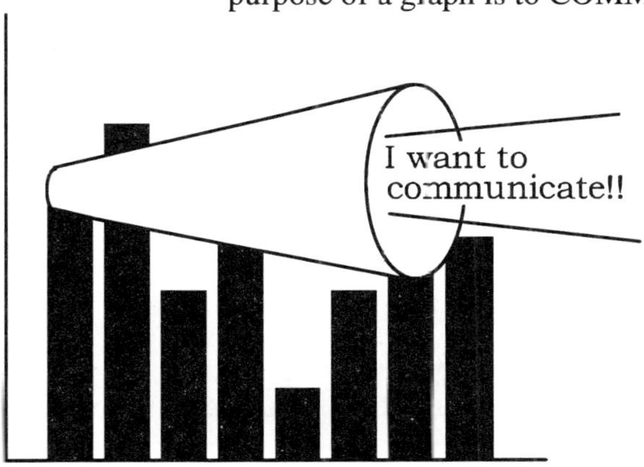

- **Right-click** on a blue column on the graph.
- **Select** 'Format Data Series'.
- **Select** [Patterns].
- **Select** 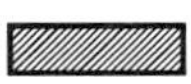 from the drop-down list of pattern options.

Hint: This the fourth from the left on the second row.

Select the black square from the colour palette.

Hint: Check that the sample box looks acceptable:

Click on OK.

3.4.5 Gridlines

In some cases, it is necessary to provide a degree of precision so that readers are able to read data values off the screen or page and where data labels would create clutter – evidence from a clinical trial would be an obvious candidate, particularly where there are a large number of data points. Gridlines can be useful in this context.

Now we can add the gridlines:

Right-click on the chart background.

Select 'Insert Gridlines'.

It is now possible to choose whether to have major or minor gridlines and to which axis they will apply.

Select Major gridlines in the Y-axis box if not already selected.

If any other gridlines are selected, de-select them by clicking on the cross in the box leaving a blank white box. When this has been done:

Click on OK.

Our graph should now look like Fig. 3.8 below.

There are numerous other ways in which graphs can be improved. Some of them will be highlighted in later chapters. The aim should be to present the information in the clearest possible way. Too much 'improvement' may lead to graphs being more complicated than necessary. So keep the graph simple!

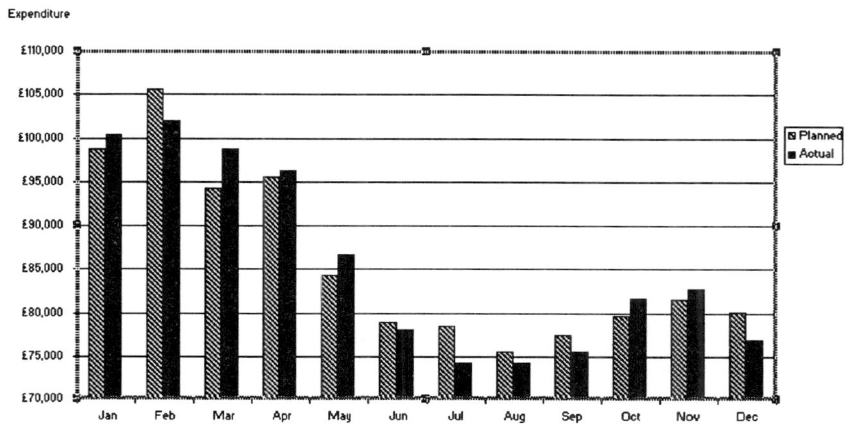

Fig. 3.8 The budget graph.

3.4.6 Printing a chart

Printing a chart is similar to printing the worksheet. When we select the Print option, the dialog box gives us three options:

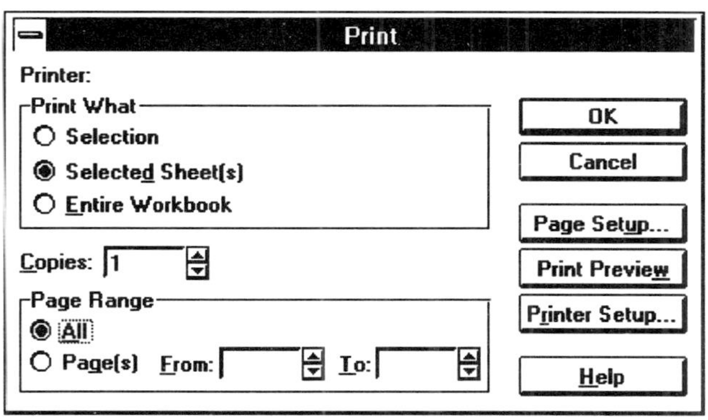

Fig. 3.9 The Print dialog box.

The default is the selected sheet, i.e. the chart.

Click on OK.

Hint: The quickest way to print the chart is simply to

☛ **Press** [Ctrl] and P together, then ↵.

or

🖱 **Click** on 🖨.

🖱 **Click** on [OK].

3.4.7 Saving your own Autoformat Styles

If you are to produce several charts, all of which are to have the same style which you have created, this is a good point at which to set the preferred style rather than using the Excel's default style. This can be done with the Autoformat feature, allowing you to define your own Autoformat style. First, we must remove any chart-specific features of our graph. In this case we should remove the customized Y-axis range:

🖱 **Right-click** on the Y-axis.

🖱 **Select** 'Format Axis'.

🖱 **Select** [Scale].

🖱 **Click** in the ☒ Minimum box.

🖱 **Click** in the ☒ Maximum box.

🖱 **Click** on [OK].

Now we can save our style using Autoformat.

🖱 **Right-click** on the chart background.

🖱 **Select** 'Autoformat'.

🖱 **Select** 'User-defined'.

🖱 **Click** on 'Customise'.

The dialog box that appears is shown in Fig. 3.10.

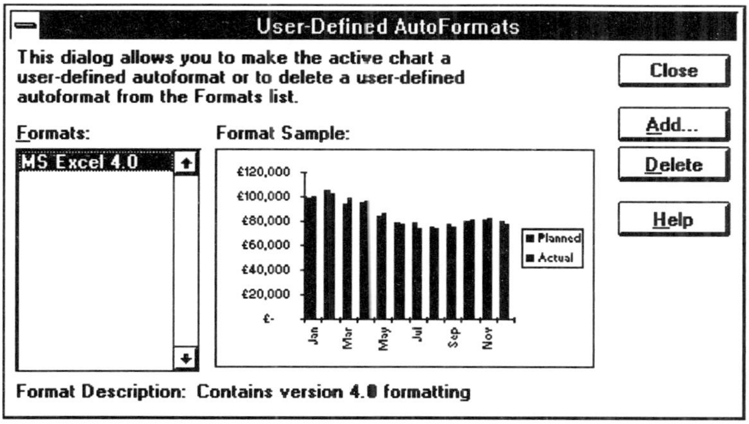

Fig. 3.10 User-defined AutoFormat dialog box.

Click on 'Add'.

Type Hatched column↵.

Click on OK.

Click on Close.

Now we can apply our user-designed Autoformat to a new chart.

Click on Sheet1 at the bottom of the sheet.

Paint cells A5 to M5.

Hold down the [Ctrl] key and **paint** A10 to M10.

Press [F11].

A new chart is created in Chart2 which is based upon the options used previously for Chart1. In order to make our chart suitable for printing in black and white we should apply our user defined Autoformat. To do this:

Right-click on the chart background.

Select 'Autoformat'.

Select 'User-defined'.

Select 'Hatched column'.

Click on OK.

The graph should now incorporate the style features of our previously defined sheet.

Now we should save the whole workbook, data and sheets together:

🖰 **Click** on [save icon] on the toolbar.

3.5 USING A PIE CHART TO REPRESENT DATA AS FRACTIONS OF THE WHOLE

3.5.1 Displaying information from the FHSA quarterly statement

There are instances where it is appropriate to show data in the form of a pie chart. In general terms, the role of the pie chart is to display the relative proportions of each piece of data as a fraction of the whole.

One specific example is where data is drawn from the quarterly return statement from the FHSA. The data will be in the form shown below. If we wish to obtain a better impression of the sources of practice income, we may create a pie chart.

Open the sheet FHSAQTR.XLS:

🖰 **Click** on [open icon].

🖰 **Select** 'fhsaqtr.xls'.

🖰 **Click** on [OK].

If we wish to depict the practice fees by category we can do so as follows:

☛ **Paint** A2:B5.

☛ **Press** [F11].

A line graph will appear in the sheet Chart 1.

🖰 **Click** on [maximize icon] to produce a full screen.

The graph can be converted to a pie as follows:

- **Right-click** on the chart background.
- **Select** 'Chart type '.

The dialog box that appears has been shown earlier in Fig.3.3.

- **Double-click** on 'Pie'.

Now use the knowledge gleaned from the last section to add a title and data labels to the pie chart. If we wish to highlight one particular component of practice income, this can be achieved by cutting that particular 'slice' from the pie. Excel highlights the largest item, in this case the standard capitation.

- **Right-click** on the chart background.
- **Select** 'Chart type'.
- **Click** on '3-D'.
- **Click** on [OK].

The pie chart can be further enhanced by the use of legends and labels in just the same manner as the line chart. It can also be saved and printed in the usual manner. We shall demonstrate the use of some other chart types, including more three-dimensional charts, as well as some more advanced features in some of the later chapters.

> **Hint:** For aesthetic reasons, a 3-D pie may be preferred. However, in terms of highlighting data a 2-D pie can be at least as effective as a 3-D pie.

4

Setting up a performance monitoring system for immunizations

4.1 CHAPTER SUMMARY

For both clinical and financial reasons, it is becoming necessary to monitor performance in primary health care. It is necessary, for example, to establish the effectiveness of preventative screening programmes in areas such as cervical cytology, child immunology, blood pressure (and so on). Amongst children, one area of great concern is the uptake of immunizations and attendance at early developmental checks. In this chapter, a system is described which will:

- monitor levels of attendance at developmental checks;
- monitor the uptake of immunizations;
- produce a quantitative performance measure.

In the process we shall introduce the following features of Excel:

- using Excel as a simple database;
- processing data as dates and fractions;
- sorting and searching data;
- logical formulae, counting entries;
- cell notes.

4.2 CHILD MONITORING SYSTEM

Excel is no substitute for a sophisticated database package but it provides some database handling functions which can be useful. We will illustrate some of these with a simple patient record system used to record child immunizations:

Open 'immune.xls'.

> **Hint:** From now on in the text we shall use the instruction 'Open' to refer to the task of opening a new sheet. This is equivalent to
>
> **Select** 'File' from the menu bar.
>
> **Select** 'Open'.
>
> **Select** 'immune.xls'.
>
> **Click** on OK.
>
> or in its briefest form
>
> **Click** on .
>
> **Double-click** on 'immune.xls'.

This is an example of an application where it is useful to have numerical and graphical functions available in a data handling application. The data sheet represents data on thirteen babies and young children concerning their birth and innoculation histories. It could be used to keep track of immunization rates in the practice. If you already have such functionality on your practice system, it can easily be amended to deal with similar problems which the practice system may not cover.

4.2.1 Using Excel as a simple database

Excel in its latest guise makes use of the concepts of data lists. A list is a column with a title in the first row and data in each of the other rows. Excel treats the first row as a header and allows you to identify the column by the text in the first row. It also ignores the first row when sorting data or carrying out similar operations. This makes using Excel as a simple database simpler than with some other spreadsheets, including previous versions of Excel.

Hint: Excel 5.0 differs radically from Excel 4.0 in this area.

The first row of the sheet Immune.xls contains a list of headers describing the data contained in each column:

Table 4.1 Lists contained in Immune.xls

Column	*Header*	*Data stored*
A	Surname:	contains the patients' surnames
B	Forenames:	contains the patients' forenames
C	Sex:	contains the patients' sex
D	DOB:	contains the patients' dates of birth
E	Birth Weight:	contains the patients' weight, stored as a fraction
F	6 week check:	contains the date that the patients attended for their 6-week check; blank indicates non-attendance
G	Triple 1	contains the date that the patients attended for their first triple immunization; blank indicates non-attendance
H	Triple 2	contains the date that the patients attended for their second triple immunization; blank indicates non-attendance
I	Triple 3	contains the date that the patients attended for their third triple immunization; blank indicates non-attendance
J	7 month check:	contains the date that the patients attended for 7-month check; blank indicates non-attendance
K	12 month MMR	contains the date that the patients attended for their MMR (Mumps, Measles and Rubella) injection at 12 months; blank indicates non-attendance

Health warning:	Excel will automatically treat data as lists providing that at least one cell is selected within the region where the data is stored. Always click on a cell before using data functions to ensure that they work correctly.

Columns D and G to K contain data in date format. To format a blank column in the same way:

Click on column L to highlight the whole column.

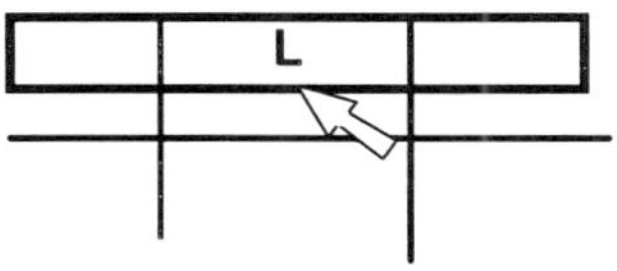

Fig. 4.1 Selecting the whole of column L.

Select 'Format' from the menu bar.

Select 'Cells'.

Select Number (if not already selected).

Select the Date Category.

Select 'dd-mmm-yy' from Format Codes.

Click on OK.

Birth weight presents a problem as it is generally recorded in pounds and ounces. This may be handled by using the fraction format. In the sheet provided column E is formatted as a fraction. If the data is input as decimals, then it is displayed as fractions allowing the ounces to appear as fractions of pounds.

To see how this was done, re-format the column L as follows:

Select 'Format' from the menu bar.

Select 'Cells'.

Select Number (if not already selected).

Select 'Fraction'.

Select '# ??/??'.

Click on [OK].

To see how this works in reality we will add some more data to complete an incomplete record: in this case, record 13, surname Gillies. Excel provides us with a form to enter our data:

Click on A2 – this could be any cell with data in it.

Select 'Data' from the menu bar.

Select 'Form'.

The form that is displayed is shown in Fig. 4.2.

The data displayed is that stored in row 2 of our sheet, because row 1 contains the header information. To add some data to our incomplete record, which is number 13, we must first find the record:

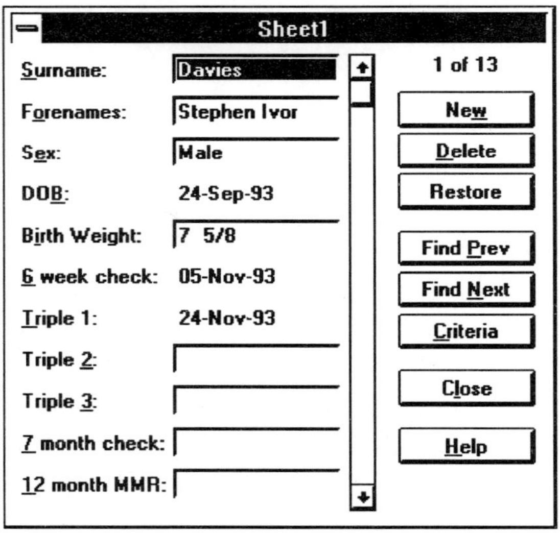

Fig. 4.2 Data entry form for record 1.

Click on 'Criteria'.

Type Gillies in the [ ] next to Surname.

Click on [Find Next].

Now we can add our data:

Click on [ ] next to Forenames.

Type Rachael Elinor ⇥.

☛ **Type** F ⇥.

☛ **Type** 7 13/16 ⇥.

The completed form should look like Fig. 4.3.

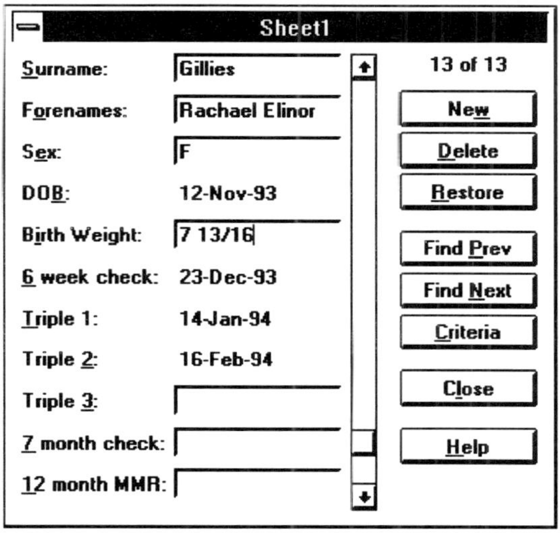

Fig. 4.3 Completed data entry form

Health warning:	Pressing ↵ before the completion of data entry will cause data entry to cease! At the completion of each box use a ⇥ (tab) key NOT a ↵ (enter) key to move to the next field. At the completion of the whole form, use a ↵ key to complete the data entry for that record

4.2.2 Sorting data

The List facility where Excel identifies each column by the label in the first row allows us to use the sort function to sort data into ascending or descending order. The sort procedure is based on the use of one or more columns as the 'key' field, identified by the label in row 1. In this particular example we shall use the Date of Birth as the key by which the records on immunizations will be sorted.

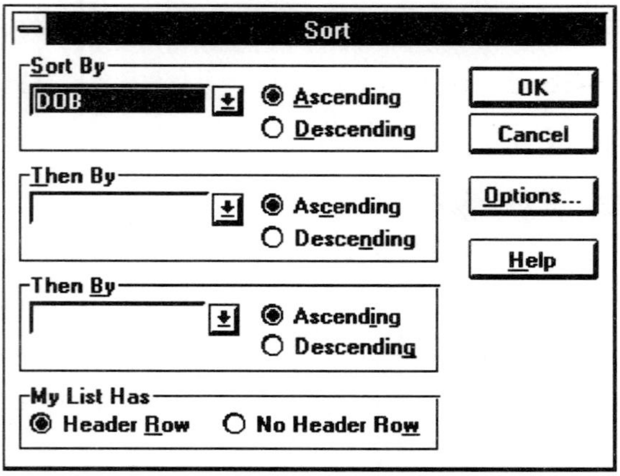

Fig. 4.4 Sort dialog box.

Click on D2.

Hint: This could be any cell in column D.

Select 'Data' from the menu bar.

Select 'Sort'.

Because we selected a cell in column D, Excel assumes that we would like to sort the data by Date of Birth. To sort, simply

Click on OK.

Hint: Remember that **Press** ↵ is always an alternative to **Click** on OK.

The records are now sorted by date of birth.

Now we shall try a more sophisticated sort where the records are sorted by Sex, Surname and Forename in that order. The records are required to be listed with boys first, then in alphabetical order of surname and then forenames. This involves the use of three keys, the order in which the columns are put in the key dialog box determining the sort order:

Select 'Data' from the menu bar.

Select 'Sort'.

Click on next to DOB in the 'Sort by' box.

From the list that appears, shown in Fig. 4.5:

Select 'Sex'.

Click on 'Descending'.

Click on in the first 'Then By' box:

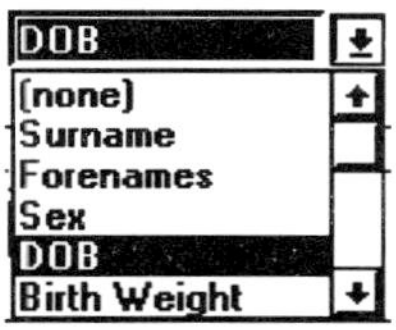

Fig. 4.5 Drop down list with list names on which to sort.

From the list that appears:

Select 'Surname'.

Click on in the second 'Then By' box.

From the list that appears,

Select 'Forenames'.

The final sort options are shown in Fig. 4.6:

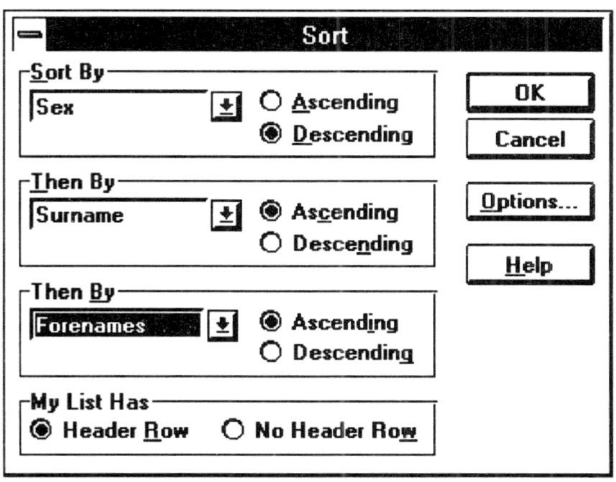

Fig. 4.6 The finished sort options for the multiple sort.

A	B	C	D	E
Surname	Forenames	Sex	DOB	Birth Weight
Brown	Paul Eliot	M	4-Jan-94	8 3/8
Davies	Stephen Ivor	M	23-Sep-93	7 5/8
Green	Nigel Henry	M	11-May-93	7 11/16
Sanderson	James Alexander	M	19-Sep-92	8 1/4
Smith	John Frederick	M	28-Feb-93	3 3/8
Smith	Robert Andrew	M	8-Feb-93	7 1/16
Burrows	Elaine	F	12-Aug-92	6 15/16
Clayton	Sara-Jane	F	10-Oct-93	7 3/16
Davis	Jennifer Susan	F	26-Mar-93	4 7/16
Gillies	Rachael Elinor	F	31-Aug-93	7 13/16
Peel	Amanda	F	3-Dec-92	6 15/16
Roberts	Andrea Jane	F	22-May-93	8 7/16
Smith	Catherine Susan	F	26-Nov-92	6 1/2

Fig. 4.7 The first five data lists after sorting.

Click on OK.

The results should look like those in Fig. 4.7.

4.2.3 Filtering data

As well as sorting data, Excel provides the facility to filter out a specific group of records. Supposing for example, we wished to select only the female children:

Click on C2.

Select 'Data' from the menu bar.

Select 'Filter'.

Select 'Autofilter'.

In the first row of each column, a appears, to signify a drop down menu.

Click on next to Sex in cell C1.

Select 'F' for female.

Only the data relating to the female patients is shown. To view only a particular patient, select their surname:

Click on ⊻ next to Surname in cell A1.

Select 'Gillies'.

If the surname does not uniquely identify a record, then we can use combinations of filters. For example to select John Smith, first restore all the data:

Click on ⊻ next to Surname in cell A1.

Select '(All)'.

Click on ⊻ next to Sex in cell C1.

Select '(All)'.

Now to select John Smith:

Click on ⊻ next to Surname in cell A1.

Select 'Smith'.

Click on ⊻ next to Forename in cell B1.

Select 'John Frederick'.

> **Hint**: With a small number of records, this operation looks unimpressive but on a list of 1,500 patients, it is much more obviously useful.

Suppose we wish to find the non-attenders for the first triple injection. We can use the (blanks) option:

First restore all the data:

Click on ⊻ next to Surname in cell A1.

Select '(All)'.

Click on ⊻ next to Forename in cell B1.

Select '(All)'.

Now to identify the non-attenders:

Click on ⊻ next to Triple1 in cell G1.

Select '(blanks)' – this is near the end of the list.

This tells us that three children have not attended for this injection. However some of these children may be too young to attend yet. To filter a set of data and specify a range of values, we use the custom criteria option. For example, to find all those children weighing over 7lbs at birth, first restore all the data:

Click on next to Triple1 in cell G1.

Select '(All)'.

Now to identify the heavier babies:

Click on next to Birth Weight in cell E1.

Select '(Custom)'.

This produces the following dialog box:

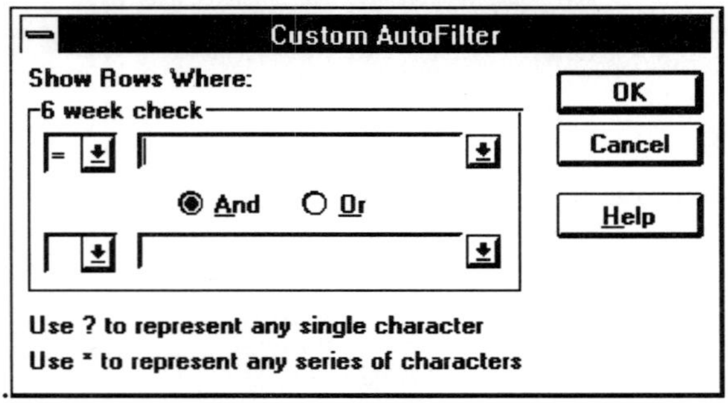

Fig. 4.8 Custom Autofilter Dialog box.

Type 7 – this corresponds to a birthweight of 7lbs.

Click on next to the = sign.

Select > – this tells the computer to select greater than 7lbs.

Click on OK.

Excel now displays those babies with birth weights greater than 7lbs. To leave Autofilter mode,

Select 'Data' from the menu bar.

Select 'Filter'.

Select 'Autofilter'.

The Autofilter facility is switched off and the drop-down menu arrows disappear.

4.2.4 Searching for and replacing data

The alternative way to find specific data is to use the search and replace facility, which works in a similar way to search and replace in a word processor. To find a cell containing a specific piece of data, say 'Ivor' we can use the Find facility. Notice that the value to be found does not have to be the whole cell value.

To find 'Ivor'

- **Click** on 'Edit' from the menu bar.
- **Click** on 'Find'.

The Find dialog box is shown in Fig. 4.9.

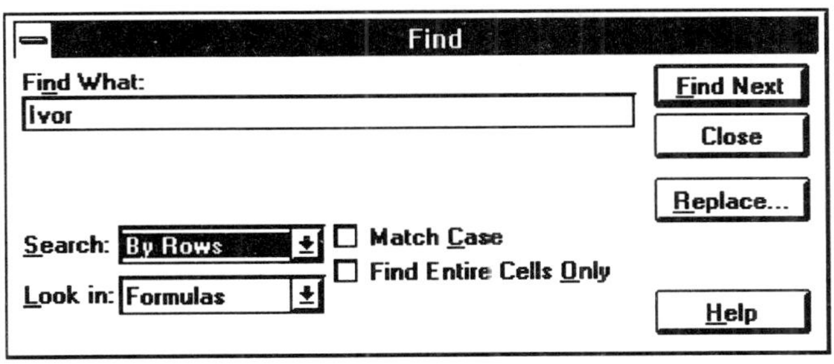

Fig. 4.9 The Find dialog box.

- **Type** Ivor↵.
- **Click** on Close.

Hint: We can use a keyboard short cut to achieve this:

- **Press** [CTRL] and F.
- **Type** Ivor↵.
- **Press** [Esc].

Hint: We can use the Find facility to find formulae and notes. This can be very helpful, since these entries are not normally displayed.

It is also possible to search for and replace data in a particular cell:

- **Click** on 'Edit'.

Click on 'Replace'.

Type M.

Hint: Typing replaces the highlighted 'Ivor'.

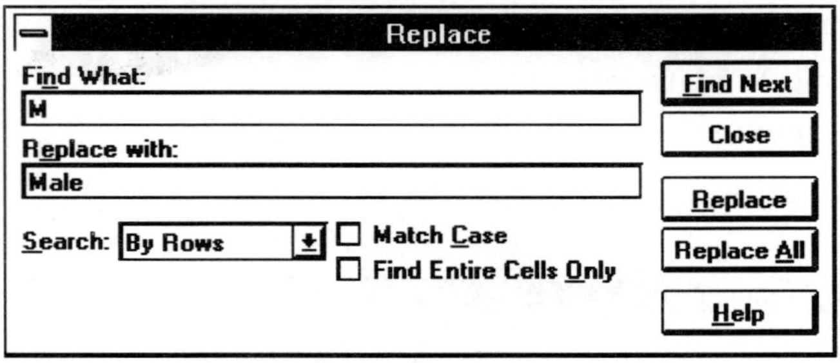

Fig. 4.10 The Replace dialog box.

Health Warning: If you miss out this stage, you will find strange values appearing like 'Maleonth'!

Click in the [box] below 'Replace with'.

At the flashing cursor in the box,

Type Male.

Click on ☐ next to 'Find Entire Cells Only'.

Click on [Find Next].

Click on [Replace All].

Now try to repeat the process yourself to substitute Female for F.

Hint: You may need to change the column width to accommodate 'Female': refer back to the last chapter if you can't remember how to do it.

4.3 PERFORMANCE MEASUREMENT

Excel is not a specialized database package, and cannot compete with packages such as Microsoft Access™ or Borland Paradox™. However, it is very good at producing quantitative measures from qualitative data and displaying these measures graphically. Thus, Excel can be a significant tool in producing quantitative performance measures.

First we shall consider some simple quantitative functions.

4.3.1 The average function

We can provide information on the average (mean) birth weight of the children with the following:

🖱 **Click** on D18.

☛ **Type** Mean.

🖱 **Click** on E18.

🖱 **Click** on [fx] (This is the Function Wizard).

The Function Wizard consists of two dialog boxes, one to select the function, the next to select the parameters, as illustrated in Fig. 4.11 overleaf. To calculate the mean birthweight:

🖱 **Select** 'Statistical' from Category if not already selected.

🖱 **Select** 'AVERAGE' from Function Name.

🖱 **Click** on [Next >]

☛ **Type** E2:E14↵.

🖱 **Click** on [Finish].

> **Hint**: It may be quicker to use the keyboard for both the last two steps:
>
> ☛ **Type** E2:E14↵.
>
> ☛ **Press** ↵.

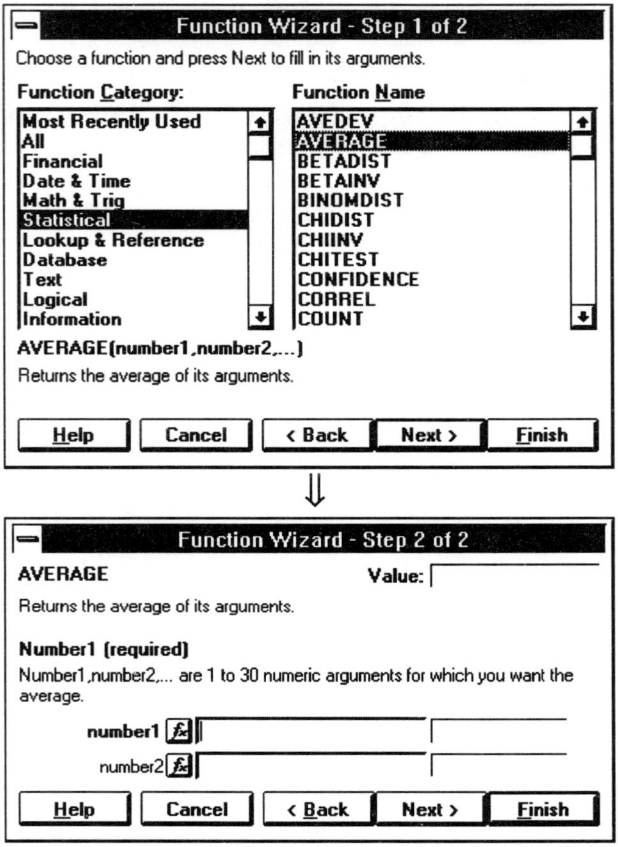

Fig. 4.11 The FunctionWizard.

Now change the format of E18 to a decimal since the fractional form no longer has significance, not being in 16ths:

Click on E18.

Select 'Format' from the menu bar.

Select 'Cells'.

Select [Number].

Select '0.00'.

Click on [OK].

The answer should be 6.97.

4.3.2 The Standard Deviation

We can go one step further in sophistication by providing some information on the dispersion of the birth weights around the average or mean value. In a large sample, we would expect 68% of the birth weights to be within plus or minus one standard deviation of the mean and 95% to be within 2 standard deviations.

- **Click** on D19.
- **Type** St.Dev.
- **Click** on E19.
- **Click** on [fx] (This is the Function Wizard).
- **Select** 'Statistical' from Function Category.
- **Select** 'STDEVP' from Function Name.

> **Hint**: The functions are listed in alphabetical order: use the scroll bar to find STDEVP; Typing S before scrolling will take you down to all the functions beginning with S

- **Click** on [Next >].
- **Type** E2:E14↵.
- **Click** on [Finish].

The answer should be 1.44. If not, see the hint on the next page!

> **Health Warning**: There are two functions for the standard deviation in Excel: STDEV and STDEVP giving the sample and population standard deviations respectively. To find out the difference, the reader is referred to D.G. Altman's book entitled 'Practical Statistics for Medical Research', published by Chapman and Hall.

> **Hint:** If the number is not showing as a decimal, then we must once again re-format the answer as a decimal:
>
> 🖱 **Click** on E19.
>
> 🖱 **Select** 'Format' from the menu bar.
>
> 🖱 **Select** 'Cells'.
>
> 🖱 **Select** [Number].
>
> 🖱 **Select** '0.00'.
>
> 🖱 **Click** on [OK].

4.3.3 Percentage of children reached

We would like to keep track of how many children are being immunized and to see what percentage of the children we are reaching. This can be done, but it is not quite as simple as it might appear. First work out how many children are being immunized or attending clinics.

🖱 **Click** on B16.

☛ **Type** Total recorded.

🖱 **Click** on C16.

🖱 **Click** on [f_x].

🖱 **Select** 'Statistical' from Function Category.

🖱 **Select** 'COUNTA'.

🖱 **Click** on [Next >]

☛ **Type** C2:C14↵.

🖱 **Click** on [Finish].

🖱 **Autofill** the formula across to K16.

Hint: To remind yourself of how Autofill works, refer back to Chapter Two.

This gives us our first measure of performance: the number of children attending for a check-up or immunization. However, performance is judged as a percentage of the total target population. This total varies according to how old the children are on any specific day.

For columns C to E, the answer is the total population, and therefore we can set these easily:

🖰 **Click** on B15.

☛ **Type** Target population.

🖰 **Click** on C15.

☛ **Type** =C16↵.

🖰 **Autofill** the formula from cell C15 across to E15.

However, whilst the total population is what was required above, this is not the case for the other columns in the table: this time it is the total population of babies who are available for checks or for immunizations. This figure will be smaller than the total population according to how many days it is from their birth date to today. For example a baby born 3 weeks ago will not be ready yet for the 6 weeks' check and therefore is not part of the population we are trying to reach with the 6 weeks' check.

In order to work out the total eligible population for F15 to K15 we must first set up a new column in L which will use a logical test to ensure that the population we seek is the one required. Effectively we shall select from all the records those where the dates of birth are more than 42 days ago (i.e. 6 weeks) in order to provide the total required population. In logical terms we say:

If today minus 42 days (i.e. 6 weeks) is greater than the birth date, place a '1' in the cell (the answer is true), otherwise place a '0' (the answer is false) in the cell.

To implement this in our sheet, we are going to use the Columns on the right of the sheet. First we must remove any spurious formatting we placed there earlier in this chapter

🖰 **Click** on the L in the column header.

- **Select** ‘Format’ from the menu bar.
- **Select** ‘Cells’.
- **Select** [Number].
- **Select** ‘All’ from Category.
- **Select** ‘General’ from Format Codes.
- **Click** on [OK].

Now we can add our formulae:

- **Click** on L2.
- **Click** on [fx].
- **Select** ‘Logical’ from Function Category.
- **Select** ‘IF’ from Function Name.
- **Click** on [Next >]

The dialog box is shown in Fig. 4.12:

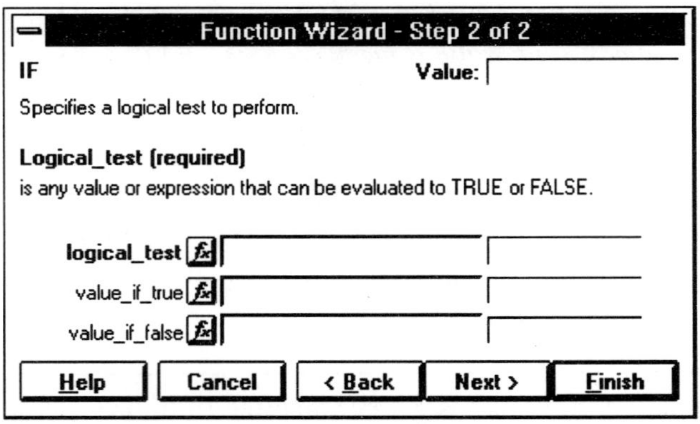

Fig. 4.12 The IF Function Wizard dialog box.

- **Type** TODAY()-42>$D2 ⇥.

> **Hint:** This is the first example of the use of an absolute reference indicated by the '$'. This means that the column reference will not change as the formula is copied across a row of cells. This has been explained in greater detail in Chapter Two.

☛ **Type** 1 ⇥.

☛ **Type** 0.

> **Hint:** The ⇥ key moves you from one data entry box to the next, without needing to use the mouse.

The completed version is shown in Fig. 4.13.

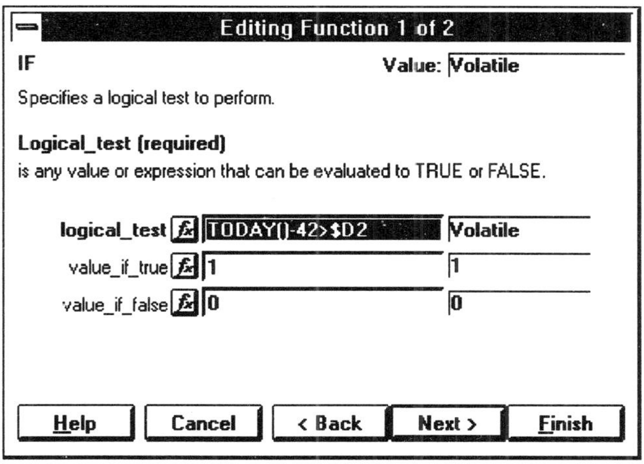

Fig. 4.13 The completed IF Function Wizard dialog box.

Once this dialog box is satisfactory,

🖱 **Click** on Finish.

The complete formula stored in cell L2 now reads:

=IF(TODAY()-42>$D2,1,0)

This is Excel's way or representing what is contained in the box. In the simplest possible terms, if the child is more than 6 weeks old, a '1' is placed in the cell, if not a '0' appears.

Hint: When the formula is completed, the value is calculated and placed in the cell. If this does not happen, then it usually means that there is an error in the formula.

- **Autofill** down the column to L14.
- **Click** on L15.
- **Click** on [Σ].
- **Click** on [☑].

Hint: This is the same as **Press** ↵.

This totals the column for you, and this represents the maximum population available for the 6 week check at today.

- **Autofill** the formula from L2 across to M2
- **Double-click** on M2.

Edit the cell from the keyboard so that the formula reads:

IF(TODAY()-$D2>62,1,0).

- **Autofill** the formula down the column to M14.
- **Click** on M15 .
- **Click** on [Σ].
- ☛ **Press** ↵.

This is the target population of children up to two months old:
Now repeat this process for columns N, O, P, Q placing

IF(TODAY()-$D2>93,1,0) in cell N2 – corresponds to 3 months ago.

IF(TODAY()-$D2>124,1,0) in cell O2 – corresponds to 4 months ago.

IF(TODAY()-$D2>217,1,0) in cell P2 – corresponds to 7 months ago.

IF(TODAY()-$D2>372,1,0) in cell Q2 – corresponds to 12 months ago.

The formulae at the end should look like the sheet illustrated in Fig. 4.14 overleaf.

Hint: If you use Autofill to copy the formula across from N2 to Q2 and edit the formulae to their appropriate values, then if you paint the cells N2 to Q2, you may Autofill the whole row down to fill the entire range of cells. This ability to Autofill a row of cells down, or a column of cells across is new in version 5.0.

L	M	N
=IF(TODAY()-42>$D2,1,0)	=IF(TODAY()-62>$D2,1,0)	=IF(TODAY()-93>$D2,1,0)
=IF(TODAY()-42>$D3,1,0)	=IF(TODAY()-62>$D3,1,0)	=IF(TODAY()-93>$D3,1,0)
=IF(TODAY()-42>$D4,1,0)	=IF(TODAY()-62>$D4,1,0)	=IF(TODAY()-93>$D4,1,0)
=IF(TODAY()-42>$D5,1,0)	=IF(TODAY()-62>$D5,1,0)	=IF(TODAY()-93>$D5,1,0)
=IF(TODAY()-42>$D6,1,0)	=IF(TODAY()-62>$D6,1,0)	=IF(TODAY()-93>$D6,1,0)
=IF(TODAY()-42>$D7,1,0)	=IF(TODAY()-62>$D7,1,0)	=IF(TODAY()-93>$D7,1,0)
=IF(TODAY()-42>$D8,1,0)	=IF(TODAY()-62>$D8,1,0)	=IF(TODAY()-93>$D8,1,0)
=IF(TODAY()-42>$D9,1,0)	=IF(TODAY()-62>$D9,1,0)	=IF(TODAY()-93>$D9,1,0)
=IF(TODAY()-42>$D10,1,0)	=IF(TODAY()-62>$D10,1,0)	=IF(TODAY()-93>$D10,1,0)
=IF(TODAY()-42>$D11,1,0)	=IF(TODAY()-62>$D11,1,0)	=IF(TODAY()-93>$D11,1,0)
=IF(TODAY()-42>$D12,1,0)	=IF(TODAY()-62>$D12,1,0)	=IF(TODAY()-93>$D12,1,0)
=IF(TODAY()-42>$D13,1,0)	=IF(TODAY()-62>$D13,1,0)	=IF(TODAY()-93>$D13,1,0)
=IF(TODAY()-42>$D14,1,0)	=IF(TODAY()-62>$D14,1,0)	=IF(TODAY()-93>$D14,1,0)
=SUM(L2:L14)	=SUM(M2:M14)	=SUM(N2:N14)

O	P	Q
=IF(TODAY()-124>$D2,1,0)	=IF(TODAY()-217>$D2,1,0)	=IF(TODAY()-372>$D2,1,0)
=IF(TODAY()-124>$D3,1,0)	=IF(TODAY()-217>$D3,1,0)	=IF(TODAY()-372>$D3,1,0)
=IF(TODAY()-124>$D4,1,0)	=IF(TODAY()-217>$D4,1,0)	=IF(TODAY()-372>$D4,1,0)
=IF(TODAY()-124>$D5,1,0)	=IF(TODAY()-217>$D5,1,0)	=IF(TODAY()-372>$D5,1,0)
=IF(TODAY()-124>$D6,1,0)	=IF(TODAY()-217>$D6,1,0)	=IF(TODAY()-372>$D6,1,0)
=IF(TODAY()-124>$D7,1,0)	=IF(TODAY()-217>$D7,1,0)	=IF(TODAY()-372>$D7,1,0)
=IF(TODAY()-124>$D8,1,0)	=IF(TODAY()-217>$D8,1,0)	=IF(TODAY()-372>$D8,1,0)
=IF(TODAY()-124>$D9,1,0)	=IF(TODAY()-217>$D9,1,0)	=IF(TODAY()-372>$D9,1,0)
=IF(TODAY()-124>$D10,1,0)	=IF(TODAY()-217>$D10,1,0)	=IF(TODAY()-372>$D10,1,0)
=IF(TODAY()-124>$D11,1,0)	=IF(TODAY()-217>$D11,1,0)	=IF(TODAY()-372>$D11,1,0)
=IF(TODAY()-124>$D12,1,0)	=IF(TODAY()-217>$D12,1,0)	=IF(TODAY()-372>$D12,1,0)
=IF(TODAY()-124>$D13,1,0)	=IF(TODAY()-217>$D13,1,0)	=IF(TODAY()-372>$D13,1,0)
=IF(TODAY()-124>$D14,1,0)	=IF(TODAY()-217>$D14,1,0)	=IF(TODAY()-372>$D14,1,0)
=SUM(O2:O14)	=SUM(P2:P14)	=SUM(Q2:Q14)

Fig. 4.14 Formulae in columns L to Q.

To transfer these values to the main table

Click on F15.

Type = L15↵.

Autofill from F15 across to K15.

Now we can work out the percentage reached:

Click on B17.

Type Percentage reached↵.

Click on C17.

Type =C16/C15↵.

Autofill to copy the formula across to K17.

With the cells still highlighted, we can change the format to a percentage:

Select 'Format' from the menu bar.

Select 'Cells'.

Select [Number].

Select 'Percentage' from Category.

Select '0%'.

The resulting figures are shown in Fig. 4.15.

Target Population	13	13	13	13	12	12	12	9	5
Total recorded	13	13	13	12	10	8	7	9	4
Percentage reached	100%	100%	100%	92%	83%	67%	58%	100%	80%

Fig. 4.15 Performance measures: cells B15 to K17.

4.3.4 Using compound formulae to simplify calculation

The previous solution uses elementary steps to arrive at a performance measure but we can combine these elementary steps to produce a more compact sheet.

To do this we can use a compound statement. First let's delete the formulae in columns L to Q:

Paint L2 to Q20.

Press [Del].

Double-click on F15.

☛ **Type** =SUM(IF(TODAY()-$D2:$D14>42,1,0)).

Health Warning: Do **not** hit the ↵ key! Instead read the next paragraph.

We are now going to make use of a compound statement. A compound statement combines two steps in one. Previously, we have used an IF statement for each record and then summed the whole column. Here we combine the two steps into one command. Remember to tell Excel that it is a compound statement by pressing [Ctrl] and [⇧] and ↵ instead of simply ↵. This must be repeated for any edits or changes. This statement also makes use of the idea of an array. An array is a group of cells to which we can apply an instruction. Thus in this case, our array is D2:D14. We have actually already used arrays in conjunction with the SUM() command alone, without drawing attention to them.

We shall revisit this idea later when we construct a frequency distribution table in the medical audit chapter.

☛ **Hold down** [Ctrl] and [⇧] and **Press** ↵.

🖱 **Autofill** the formulae across to K15.

🖱 **Double-click** on G15.

☛ Change the figure 42 to 62 by typing at the keyboard.

☛ **Hold down** [Ctrl]and [⇧] and **Press** ↵.

🖱 **Double-click** on H15.

☛ Change the figure 42 to 93 by typing at the keyboard.

☛ **Hold down** [Ctrl]and [⇧] and **Press** ↵.

🖱 **Double-click** on I15.

☛ Change the figure 42 to 124 by typing at the keyboard.

☛ **Hold down** [Ctrl]and [⇧] and **Press** ↵.

🖱 **Double-click** on J15.

☛ Change the figure 42 to 217 by typing at the keyboard.

☛ **Hold down** [Ctrl]and [⇧] and **Press** ↵.

🖱 **Double-click** on K15.

☛ Change the figure 42 to 372 by typing at the keyboard

☛ **Hold down** [Ctrl]and [⇧] and **Press** ↵.

4.4 ENHANCING THE SYSTEM

4.4.1 Keeping notes

The information shown in an individual cell may not tell the whole tale. It is possible to add notes to each of the cells in the sheet to provide more explanation:

🖱 **Click** on G9, the cell relating to the first triple for Sara Jane Clayton.

🖱 **Select** 'Insert' from the menu bar.

🖱 **Select** 'Note'.

☛ **Type** a note, e.g. spoke to parent: objected to immunization.

🖱 **Click** on [OK].

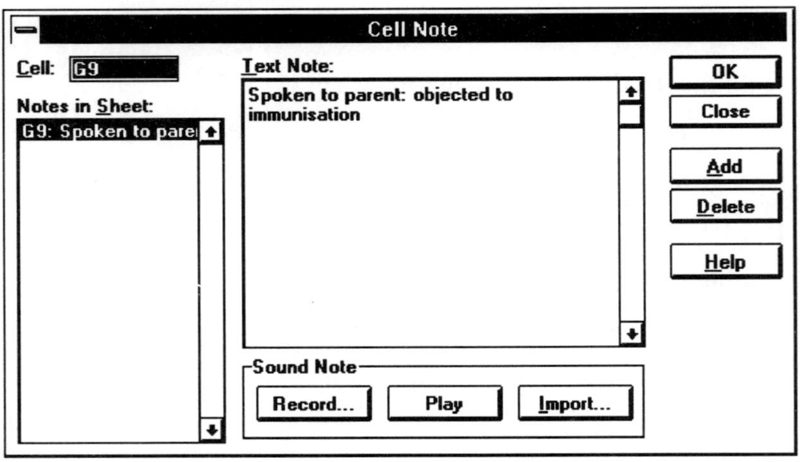

Fig. 4.16 Cell note dialog box.

If the note indicator option is selected, a red square appears in the top right-hand corner of the cell to show that a note is present: . If you wish to read the note behind the cell, then you can either repeat the above or:

- Press [⇧] and F2.

> **Hint**: If the note indicator option is switched off, we select 'Options' to show where notes are added to cells:
>
> - **Select** 'Tools' from the menu bar.
> - **Select** 'Options'.
> - **Click** on [View] if not already at the front.
> - **Click** on ☐ next to 'Note Indicator'.
> - **Click** on [OK].

From the dialog box notes can be subsequently added and deleted.

- **Select** 'Close' to return to the sheet.

Very often, the same note may crop up in different cells. For example in this case, we may wish to include the same note in cells H12 and I12. To do this:

- **Click** on G9.
- **Click** on .
- **Paint** cells H9 and I9.
- **Select** 'Edit' from the menu bar.
- **Select** 'Paste Special'.
- **Click** on 'Notes' from the Paste list.
- **Click** on [OK].
- **Press** [Esc] to remove outline marquee.

The note is now attached to each of the three cells and the note indicator should appear in all three.In these days of multimedia, Excel will even store spoken notes!

4.4.2 Adding the date and time to a sheet

It is sometimes useful to show when a sheet was actually produced and printed. We shall add the date and time to the sheet.

- **Click** on A18.
- **Click** on [fx].
- **Select** 'Date & Time' from the Function Category.
- **Select** 'NOW()' (gives today's date) from Function Name.
- **Click** on [Finish].

This gives today's date and time.

- **Autofill** the formula across to B18.
- **Click** on A18.
- **Select** 'Format' from the menu bar.
- **Select** 'Cells'.
- **Select** [Number].
- **Select** 'Date' from Category.
- **Select** 'dd-mmm-yy' from Format Codes **.**
- **Click** on [OK].
- **Click** on B18.
- **Select** 'Format' from the menu bar.
- **Select** 'Cells'.
- **Select** 'Time' from Category.
- **Select** 'hh:mm AM/PM' from Format Codes.
- **Click** on [OK].

Each time the sheet is used and printed today's date and time will be displayed. Many other things can be done with date and time to undertake scheduling and planning work.

5

Forecasting and estimating

5.1 CHAPTER SUMMARY

Forecasting and estimating are difficult tasks. For example, you may have been asked to predict the cost of drugs prescribed by your practice over the next year. Historical data is available for 10 previous quarters. A forecast for the next four is required and must be justified to colleagues. You may be involved in basic research or clinical trials analysis where estimates of relationships between variables are required as the basis for a research paper or report.

The problems covered in this chapter include:

- the derivation of a general strategy for forecasting;
- forecasting financial expenditure for the coming year;
- regression and correlation analysis used in medical research.

Excel features covered in this chapter include:

- use of Autofill for simple forecasting;
- use of scenarios and goal seeking;
- correlation analysis to find associations between variables;
- regression analysis to estimate relationships between variables.

5.2 EXCEL AND FORECASTING

Excel has a variety of statistical routines which can be used to help analyse these issues. It is not the aim here, however, to examine the statistical methods themselves. A good introduction to these issues may be found in Douglas G. Altman 'Practical Statistics for Medical Research' (Chapman & Hall, 1991). The use of forecasting will become an important part of practice planning. Excel is a good tool for forecasting trends as it combines good graphics with sophisticated tools for forecasting.

5.3 A FORECASTING STRATEGY

Forecasting is a dangerous business at the best of times (just ask any meteorologist). Central to the production of realistic budgets is the process of estimation and planning. Apart from 'guesstimates' and the use of witchcraft or divine revelation, forecasts of the future must be based on knowledge of past events. In order to carry out any estimation of sales of a product over a period of time, we need a strategy for forecasting - a series of steps undertaken to ensure that a reasonable forecast is derived from the historical data.

The steps in this strategy are as follows:

- visual inspection of the data;
- analysis;
- prediction;
- judgement.

5.3.1 Visual inspection of the data

The first stage in this analysis involves visual inspection of the data. In the sheet, Pact.xls, there are six sets of data covering 10 periods - in this case, quarters of the year. Generally, annual data may prove to be least useful in that, over 10 periods, data in years stretches over too long a period for accurate prediction. On the other hand, data in months may involve too short a time period, particularly where seasonality is involved.

Data in quarters can cover a long enough time period and can capture the seasonal variations in the data. Exactly what interval is used will very much depend on the circumstances. Load the Pact data by:

- **Open** the sheet PACT.XLS.

First, we may simply plot all the data in a single chart in an attempt to get an overall impression of the data.

- **Paint** A2 to K7.
- **Select** 'Insert' from the menu bar.
- **Select** 'Chart'.
- **Select** 'As new sheet'.
- Using the ChartWizard, create the graph shown in Fig. 5.1.

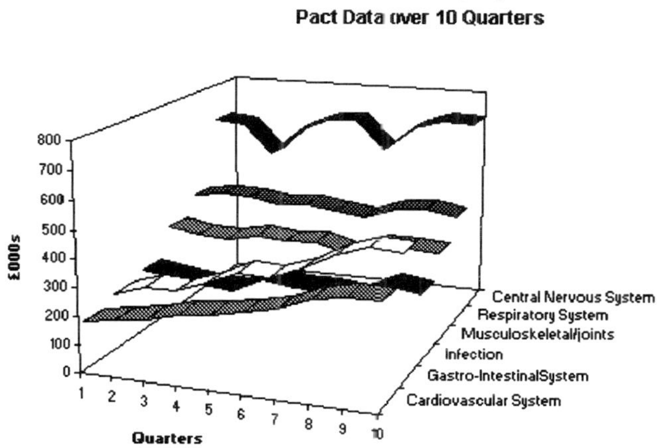

Fig. 5.1 Chart to facilitate visual analysis of data.

Visual inspection can be vital to see if predictions are sensible. In this first stage we should select that data series which looks capable of analysis. Data which appears highly random is unlikely to be capable of prediction. If we take the data above, it should be possible to forecast future prescribing costs for the Cardiovascular System. However, the degree of information obtainable from an overall plot is limited. Use the ChartWizard to draw a line graph for the Cardiovascular System data only:

- Click on PACT1 tab to return to the worksheet.

- **Paint** B2 to K2.
- **Select** 'Insert' from the menu bar.
- **Select** 'Chart'.
- **Select** 'As new sheet'.

Follow the steps shown previously to create a graph similar to that in Fig. 5.2.

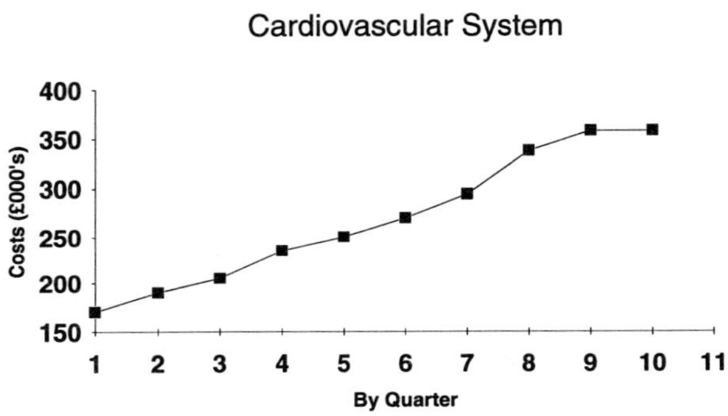

Fig. 5.2 Line graph of a single data series.

5.3.2 Analysis

The graph suggests that there is an upward trend in the data which should allow forecasting to take place. Visual inspection should be tempered, however, with knowledge of known cost movements and assessment of the impact of factors such as FHSA or Government policy changes.

5.3.3 Prediction

The easiest way to start the forecast process is to use Autofill which makes the best estimate it can for a trend. The results produced are generally reasonable:

- **Autofill** across from K1 to M1 to add extra labels. Note that Autofill correctly interprets Qtr1 as part of a series.
- **Paint** B2 to K2 – the row containing costs for Cardiovascular.
- **Autofill** across from the end of the painted range as far as M2.

Excel will fill in the values for L2 and M2 on the basis of the values in B3:K3. The predicted figures for cardiovascular system prescribing costs for the next two quarters are (to two decimal places):

	A	B
1	Qtr2	Qtr3
2	391.13	413.74

Fig. 5.3 Results of prediction by Autofill.

Now the data including the forecast for the next two quarters can be graphed using the ChartWizard. Extend the highlighted cell range as follows:

- **Hold down** the [⇧] key and **drag** the mouse from the existing painted area in row 2 up to row 1 to include the labels.

Use the ChartWizard to create a new graph containing the predicted result. The last two data points on the graph are the predicted values for the next two quarters. These may be highlighted using the Data Labels Option referred to previously. The finished workbook is available for comparison as PACT1.XLS.

5.3.4 Judgement

There are a variety of ways in which we can add to the analysis and form differing judgements of the predicted turnouts. This can involve the use of statistical techniques to help form a judgement. The use of such techniques is beyond the scope of this book. However, judgement can be formed allowing for many qualitative factors not easily amenable to statistical analysis – factors such as policy changes will have a bearing on the predicted outcomes. These must be allowed for in using the outputs of powerful statistical packages.

5.4 SCENARIOS

Forming a judgement can be aided by some of the facilities available in Excel. Imagine a three-partner practice in which the partners are discussing the budget plans over the next year. There will be differing views as to how budgets will be managed and issues regarding the ability of the practice to stay within its budgets for the year. Certain facilities in the Excel spreadsheet allow the partners to explore the situation in some detail and ensure that discussion will be enlightened by some information in order to help come to a sound judgement. A budget sheet similar but not identical to the budget sheet completed earlier will be used to demonstrate the principles.

🖰 **Open** 'budget3.xls'.

The main difference between this and the previous sheet is that:

- all the planned figures are currently blank;
- there is a small area in the top left corner of the sheet which has a scenario.

Cell B3, which is blank, will contain the initial monthly budget; cell B4 will contain the annual growth rate in the planned budget. The planned figures from January to December will be generated from these initial figures. For planning purposes this makes the current sheet more versatile than the original sheet since various scenarios can be built up showing different combinations of initial figures and their impact on the total budget for the year.

We shall now fill in the blank area of the sheet.

🖰 **Click** on B3.

☛ **Type** '95000' – this is the initial monthly budget.

🖰 **Click** on B4.

☛ **Type** '5' – this is the annual % growth rate.

Click on B11.

Type '=B3'↵.

The January figure will be the same as the initial monthly budget figure. However, we do not enter the actual figure of 95000. We draw it off the scenario panel.

Click on C11.

The February figure will be equal to January's plus one twelfth of the annual growth:

Type '=B11*(1+$B$4/1200)'↵.

Make sure that the reference to B4 is absolute (i.e. $) as the growth rate only appears in this cell.

> **Hint**: The reason for the above being divided by 1200 rather than 12 is that the percentage in B4 needs to be expressed as a proportion of the figure in B11. The alternative in B4 would have been to enter the percentage as a proportion i.e. 0.05 instead of 5%.

Autofill from C11across to M11.

The months January to December are now complete with the total, previously calculated, also available. The benefit of this approach is that we can now change the figures in B3 and B4 in order to see what impact there is on the overall budget position. With a spreadsheet set up in this manner, it is not always easy to see what the impact is of each change made in the figures. They also have to be recorded each time. The partners in the practice may well have different views about the budget turnout. It would be useful to record them separately. This can be done using the Scenario Manager.

Ensure that the cursor is located over column N where the totals are located and that the Totals column is over to the left-hand side of the screen.

Select 'Tools' from the menu bar.

Select 'Scenarios'.

The Scenario Manager, as shown below in Fig. 5.4, will now appear on the right-hand side of the screen.

Hint: You may have to drag the Scenario box across the screen in order to view column N.

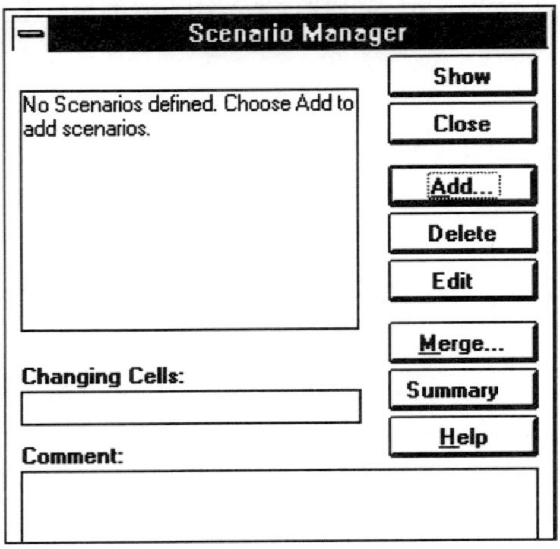

Fig. 5.4 The Scenario Manager dialog box.

Click on Add

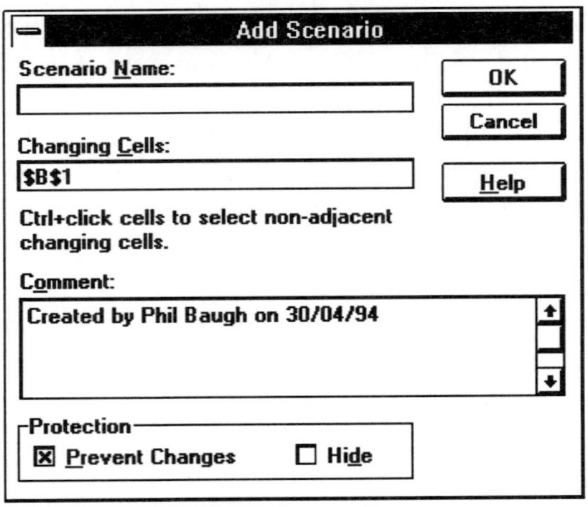

Fig. 5.5 The Add Scenario dialog box.

Imagine that Dr Green, one of the practice partners, considers a scenario where the initial monthly budget is £94000 and the growth rate is 4%. We can now add Dr Green's scenario, as shown in Fig. 5.5.

- **Type** 'Dr Green' in the 'Scenario Name' Box.
- **Type** ' B3:B4' in the 'Changing Cells' Box.

Remember that these cells contain the initial monthly budget and % growth figures.

- **Click** on OK.

The current value for each cell will now be shown as in Fig.5.6.

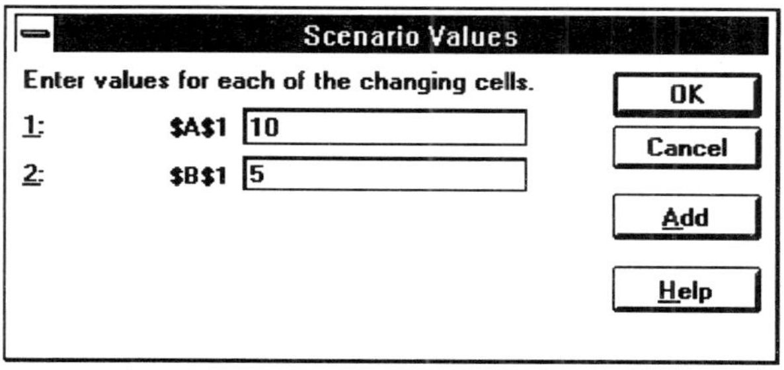

Fig. 5.6 The Scenario Values dialog box.

- **Type** ' 94000' instead of 95000 in cell B3.
- **Type** '4' instead of 5 in cell B4.
- **Click** on OK.

We can now repeat the process for the other two practice partners Dr Brown and Dr White:

	B3	B4
Dr Brown's Scenario	96000	6
Dr White's Scenario	95500	5.5

Fig. 5.7 Values entered for the partners' scenarios.

Now we can investigate the effect of each of these scenarios. Within the Scenario Manager:

- **Click** on 'Dr Green' in the Scenario Name dialog box.

Click on Show.

This will now show the effect of inputting this scenario on the totals column as the sheet is recalculated from the beginning with the new scenario values. Repeat the process for the Scenarios for Dr Brown and Dr White to see the several effects.

Click on Close.

Return to the top left of the spreadsheet. You will see that the figures from the last scenario calculated will be shown in the Scenario panel. Now input the original figures in Cells B3 and B4. (£95000 and 5%). Whilst observing the changes made by using the Scenario Manager is useful, the planning process can be enhanced by producing a summary of the changes.

Click on 'Tools' from the menu bar.

Click on 'Scenarios'.

Click on Summary within the Scenario Manager.

Scenario Summary should be highlighted. If it is not click on the circle next to the title.

Delete any references in the 'Results Cell' box.

Type 'N11,N14,N16'.

Click on OK.

These cells contain the total planned budget, the total variance and the total % variance. These will be shown in the scenario summary when the worksheet has been re-calculated. After a few seconds a new sheet will appear called Scenario Summary as shown in Fig 5.8 giving the results from the original values (called current values) and from the scenarios of the three practice partners.

Scenario Summary					
		Current Values:	Dr Green	Dr Brown	Dr White
Changing Cells:					
	$B$3	£ 95,000.00	£ 96,000.00	£ 94,000.00	£ 95,500.00
	$B$4	5	6	4	5.5
Result Cells:					
	$N$11	£ 1,166,491	£ 1,184,214	£ 1,148,912	£ 1,175,335
	$N$14	£8,372.27	£26,094.99	(-£9,207.49)	£17,215.69
	$N$16	0.7%	2.2%	(-0.8%)	1.5%

Notes: Current Values column represents values of changing cells at time Scenario Summary Report was created. Changing cells for each scenario are highlighted in gray.

Fig. 5.8 The results shown in the Scenaric Summary worksheet.

The sheet looks rather different from previous sheets with plus and minus boxes at the top and left-hand side. Experiment with clicking on these signs which will cause portions of the results to disappear and re-appear. Hiding parts of the summary can be useful for discussion purposes.

5.5 GOAL SEEKING

Another useful way of approaching the budgeting problem is to use goal-seeking techniques. One of the partners may state that what is important at the end-of-year is not the figure showing by how much the actual budget deviates from the planned budget but finding out what the initial monthly budget figure or the percentage growth rate must be in order to ensure that the budget balances at the year-end. This is the process of goal seeking starting at a result and asking what the initial condition must be.

Goal seeking can only operate on one variable at a time. If we asked the question what happens if we want to balance the budget by both altering the initial monthly budget and the percentage growth rate, then we would find that there is an infinite number of solutions. We shall therefore commence by examining the changes on the initial monthly budget. First, return to 'sheet1'. Then:

- **Click** on B3.
- **Select** 'Tools' from the menu bar.
- **Select** 'Goal Seek'.

A Goal Seek dialog box will appear.

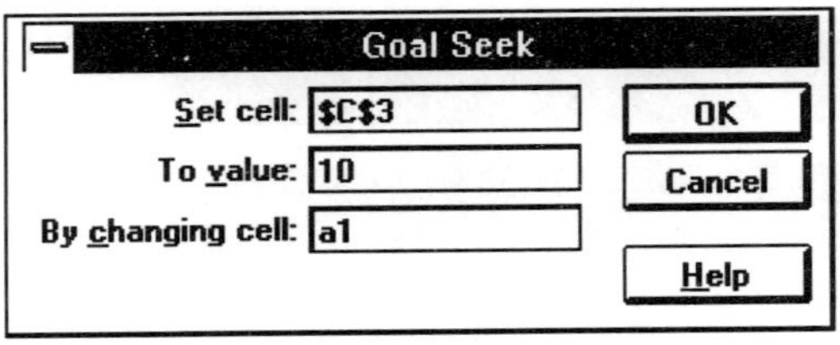

Fig. 5.9 The Goal Seek dialog box.

- **Type** 'N14' in the 'Set Cell' Box - this contains the total budget variance.
- **Type** '0' in the 'To value' box.
- **Type** 'B3' in the 'By changing cell' box.
- **Click** on OK.

After a few seconds a Goal Seek Status box as shown below will appear and will soon indicate that a solution has been found.

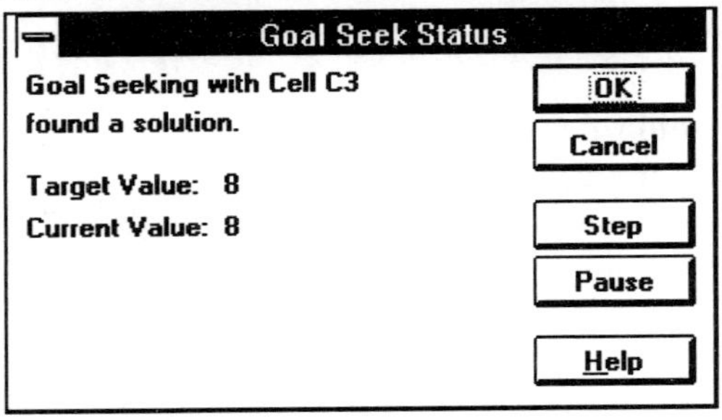

Fig. 5.10 The solution found with target and current values equal.

- **Click** on OK.

The value £94,318 can be seen in cell B3. Examination of cell N14 will show that there is no total budget variance. Change the figure in cell B3 back to £95, 000 and repeat the operation, this time for the percentage growth.

- **Select** 'Tools' from the menu bar.
- **Select** 'Goal Seek'.

☛ **Type** 'N14' in the 'Set Cell' box - this contains the total budget variance.

☛ **Type** ' 0' in the 'To value' box.

☛ **Type** ' B4' in the 'By changing' box.

🖰 **Click** on OK.

The Goal Seek Status box will soon appear.

🖰 **Click** on OK.

This time the value of 3.43% (to two decimal places) will be found in cell B4. Goal seeking is a very powerful method for examining budgets. Although a simple model has been developed here, much more complex budgetary models are also amenable to this form of analysis.

5.6 CORRELATION ANALYSIS

For research and clinical trial purposes we need to go a great deal further than has been described up to this point. Correlation analysis is a means to analyze the association between two or more variables. To begin with, we shall examine the association between just two variables: age and the percentage of body weight stored as fat. It might be expected that as age increases so does the percentage of body weight stored as fat. Later, we shall introduce a further variable, the sex of the sample individuals, to highlight potential problems with this type of analysis. Using the example from Mazess *et al.* quoted in Altman (*op.cit.*), a correlation between the two variables can be shown. As before, the first stage in the analysis is visual inspection of the data.

We shall use the worksheet, agebody.xls, to analyze the data which is shown below in Table 5.1.

🖰 **Open** 'agebody.xls'.

🖰 **Paint** B1 to C19.

🖰 **Select** 'Insert' from the menu bar.

🖰 **Select** 'Chart'.

🖰 **Select** 'As new sheet'.

Click on Next > as the data is as required.

Table 5.1 Data for correlation example

Subject	*Age*	*%Fat*	*Sex*
1	23	9.5	M
2	23	27.9	F
3	27	7.8	M
4	27	17.8	M
5	39	31.4	F
6	41	25.9	F
7	45	27.4	M
8	49	25.2	F
9	50	31.1	F
10	53	34.7	F
11	53	42	F
12	54	29.1	F
13	56	32.5	F
14	57	30.3	F
15	58	33	F
16	58	33.8	F
17	60	41.1	F
18	61	34.5	F

Click on 'XY (Scatter)'.

Click on Next >.

Select 'Format1' which shows data points only.

Click on Next > twice to show Step 5.

Click on 'No' to legend as this is not necessary for a scatter plot where both axes will be labelled. Now add in a title for the chart.

Type 'Association between Age and % Body Fat' for the Chart Title .

Type 'Age' – for the X-axis Title.

Type '% Body Fat' – for the Y-axis Title.

Click on Finish.

The result is illustrated in Fig.5.11. As the graph shows, there is some degree of association between the two variables but that it is not very strong. We can now measure the strength of that association by using the Pearson correlation coefficient.

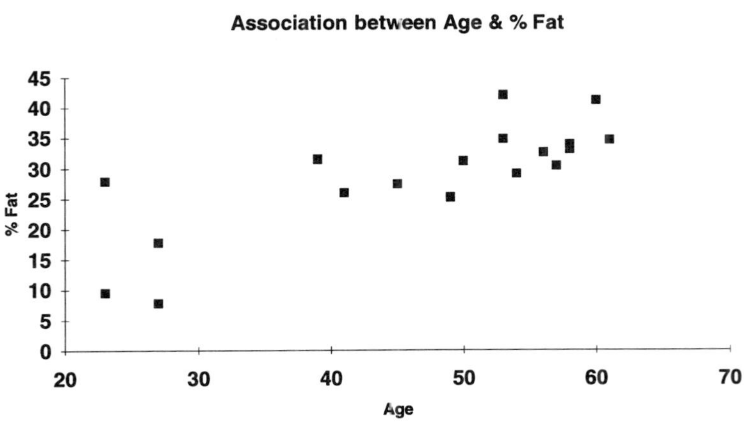

Fig. 5.11 Scatter plot of relationship between age and percentage of fat.

Return to the Agebody sheet:

Click on E2.

Type r= – r denotes the correlation co-efficient.

Click on F2.

Click on f_x.

Select 'Statistical' from Function Category.

Select 'Correl' from Function Name.

Click on Next >.

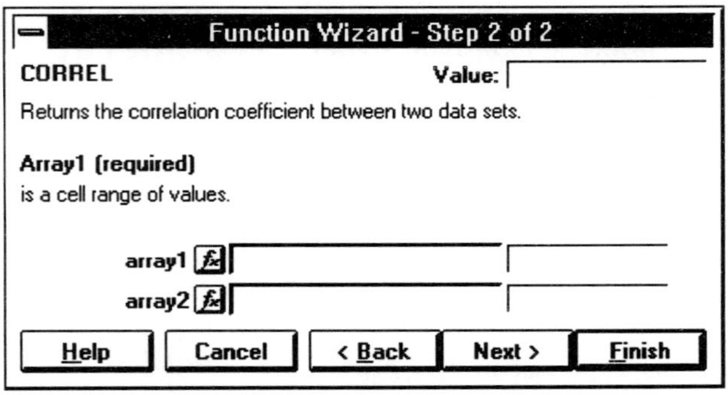

Fig. 5.12 The Correlation dialog box under the CORREL() function.

In the Correlation dialog box two arrays are asked for. (An array is simply a row or column of data.)

Type B2:B19 for the first array.

Press ⇥ to move to the second array.

Type C2:C19 for the second array.

Click on Finish.

The result will be shown on the highlighted cell: 0.792086. The value of the correlation coefficient varies between -1 and +1 where 0 indicated no statistical association, +1 indicated a strong positive association and -1 indicates a strong negative association. In this case we have a strong(ish) association. An alternative method to the above is to use the Data Analysis option from the Tools menu:

- **Select** 'Tools' from the command bar.
- **Select** 'Data Analysis'.

You will have to wait while this part of the package is loaded.

- **Select** 'Correlation'.
- **Click** on OK.

A different Correlation dialog box will now appear, as shown in Fig. 5.13.

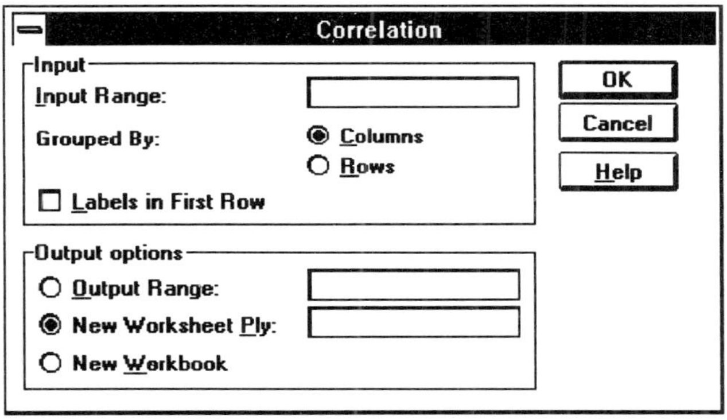

Fig. 5.13 The Correlation dialog box under the Data analysis tools.

- **Type** B2:C19 for the Input Range.
- **Select** Output Range for the output option rather than sending the results to another sheet.
- **Type** the cell reference for the beginning of an area of empty cells e.g. G5.
- **Click** on OK.

After a few seconds, the output will be shown as a table in the following style:

Table 5.2 Results of data analysis option.

	Column 1	*Column 2*
Column 1	1	
Column 2	0.792086	1

This approach to correlation using the Data Analysis option is most useful when there are a number of variables to be examined. A matrix as shown above will be created showing correlations between all variables. However, this example does also illustrate one of the pitfalls of this kind of analysis. To see the problem we must first sort our patients according to sex:

- **Paint** A1:D19.
- **Select** 'Data' from the menu bar.
- **Select** 'Sort'.
- **Click** on next to Subject in the 'Sort By' box.

From the list that appears:

- **Select** 'Sex'.

The Sort dialog box should now look like Fig. 5.14:

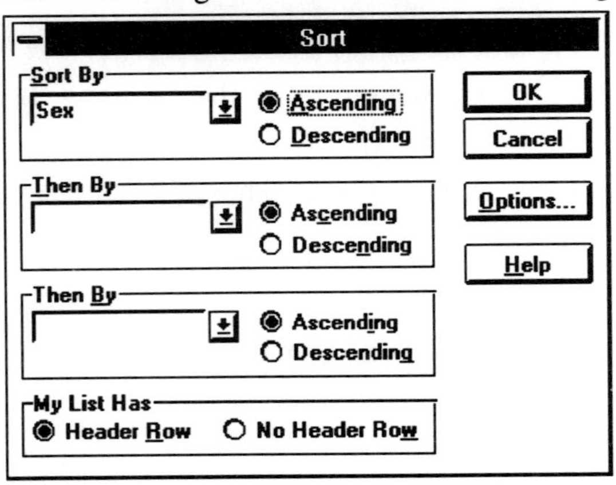

Fig. 5.14 Sort dialog box.

- **Click** on OK.

Now we can easily find the correlation coefficient for the male and female patients:

- **Click** on E4.
- **Type** 'r (F)='.
- **Click** on F4.
- **Click** on f_x.
- **Select** 'Statistical' from Function Category.
- **Select** 'Correl' from Function Name.
- **Click** on Next >.
- **Type** B2:B15 for the first array.
- **Type** C2:C15 for the second array.
- **Click** on Finish.
- **Paint** E4 to F4.
- **Click** on the Copy button.
- **Paint** E5 to F5.
- **Click** on the Paste button.
- **Click** on E5.
- **Edit** the cell so that it reads 'r(M)='.
- **Click** on F5.
- **Edit** the formula so that it reads '=CORREL(B16:B19,C16:C19)'.

The completed sheet is now shown in Fig. 5.15.

The correlation coefficient for female patients is now 0.51, much lower than for the whole sample. The male figure derived from only four patients is 0.89. Men have a lower percentage of their body weight as fat than women. Because the men in this sample happened to be younger, the mixed sample appeared more strongly linked than is the case. Thus the small and skewed sample gave a spurious credibility to the relationship. A larger sample will tend to randomize other factors and therefore produce a more reliable result.

	A	B	C	D	E	F
1	Subject	Age	%Fat	Sex		
2	2	23	27.9	F	r=	0.792086
3	5	39	31.4	F		
4	6	41	25.9	F	r(F)=	0.506589
5	8	49	25.2	F	r(M)=	0.890781
6	9	50	31.1	F		
7	10	53	34.7	F		
8	11	53	42	F		
9	12	54	29.1	F		
10	13	56	32.5	F		
11	14	57	30.3	F		
12	15	58	33	F		
13	16	58	33.8	F		
14	17	60	41.1	F		
15	18	61	34.5	F		
16	1	23	9.5	M		
17	3	27	7.8	M		
18	4	27	17.8	M		
19	7	45	27.4	M		

Fig. 5.15 Results of correlation analysis.

5.7 REGRESSION

Regression analysis is useful when there is a need to describe the relationship between one dependent variable and one or more independent variables and assess by how much the value of a dependent variable will change in response to changes in the independent variables. In order to illustrate the issues and the way in which we can use the Excel regression features we shall look at the case of the effect of fasting blood glucose (Fbg) on the mean velocity of circumferential shortening of the left ventricle (Vcf) for type 1 diabetic patients. The data is from Thuesen *et al* (1985) as used in Altman (*op.cit.*). Fbg is measured in mmol per litre and Vcf in % per second. The data is shown in Table 5.3.

Table 5.3 Data for the regression example

Patient	Fbg (mmol/l)	Vcf (%/sec)	Patient	Fbg	Vcf
1	15.3	1.76	13	19	1.95
2	10.8	1.34	14	15.1	1.28
3	8.1	1.27	15	6.7	1.52
4	19.5	1.47	16	4.2	1.12
5	7.2	1.27	17	10.3	1.37
6	5.3	1.49	18	12.5	1.19
7	9.3	1.31	19	16.1	1.05
8	11.1	1.09	20	13.3	1.32
9	7.5	1.18	21	4.9	1.03
10	12.2	1.22	22	8.8	1.12
11	6.7	1.25	23	9.5	1.7
12	5.2	1.19			

Open 'glucose.xls'.

As in the previous example, visual inspection is the first step in the process. It is important to assess whether there is any visible association between the variables. A scatter diagram is therefore appropriate.

Paint B3:C25.

Select 'Insert' from the menu bar.

Select 'Chart'.

Select 'As new sheet'.

Click on [Next >] as the data is as required.

Select 'XY Scatter' – the preferred graph.

Click on [Next >].

Select 'Format1' – the preferred format.

Click on [Next >] twice.

Select 'No' for the legend as the axis titles will show the labels for the two variables.

Click on the Title box to insert the title.

Type 'Relationship between Fbg and Vcf'.

Click on the X-axis title.

Type 'Fbg (mmol/l)'.

Click on the Y-axis title.

Type 'Vcf (%/sec)'.

Click on [Finish].

The graph will now be drawn but the scale of the Y-axis starts at 0 which tends to show the data points close together as they are distributed between Vcf values of 1.0 and 2.0. The Y-axis scale can be changed:

Double-click on the Y-axis to produce a white square at either end and to bring up the menu.

Click on Scale .

Type 0.8 in the 'Minimum Value' box.

Note that the cross in the 'Auto' box disappears – automatic scaling is switched off by inserting a figure in the 'Minimum Value' box.

Click on OK .

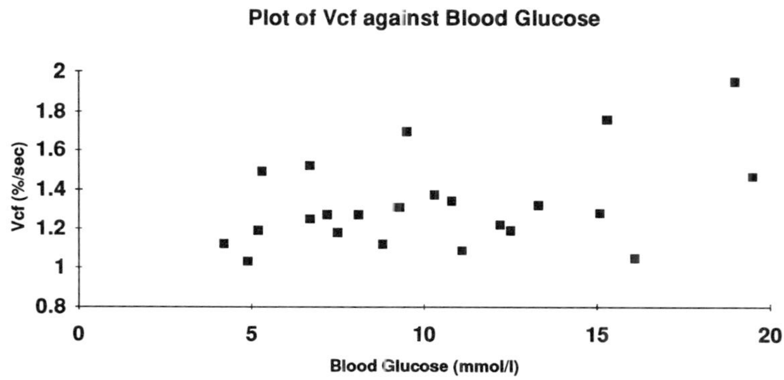

Fig. 5.16 The scatter plot.

The diagram as shown above will now show the data points more spread out than before. With inspection of the data it is now a question of whether to proceed. It is obvious that there is not a strong relationship. There may be other variables which may influence the value of Vcf. However, it may be worth examining the strength of the relationship of Fbg to Vcf at this stage. Using regression analysis we shall be able to estimate the effect any particular level of Fbg has on the rate of Vcf and by how much the Vcf rate may change in response to a change in the level of Fbg.

In Excel there are two methods by which we may do this – one of which produces limited results and the other which produces comprehensive results.

5.7.1 Method 1

Method 1 uses the LINEST function from the Function Wizard. LINEST is the regression analysis function within the Function Wizard which will produce a linear estimate. Return to the data sheet:

- **Click** on D3.
- **Click** on [fx].
- **Select** 'Statistical'.
- **Select** 'Linest'.
- **Click** on [Next >].
- **Select** 'Known y's' – these are the values of the dependent variable, Vcf.
- **Type** C$3:C$25.
- **Select** 'Known x's' – these are the values of the independent variable, Fbg.
- **Type** B$3:B$25.
- **Click** on 'Const'.
- **Type** 1 (the word true will appear in the right hand box to indicate that we require a constant in the estimate).
- **Click** on [Finish].

The answer that appears is 0.021963. This is the value of the m co-efficient, or the gradient of the line of best fit. To calculate the intercept value and thus define the line of best fit uniquely:

- **Autofill** down from D3 to D4.
- **Click** on D4.
- **Click** between the '=' and the 'L' in the edit bar.
- **Type** INDEX(.

☛ **Press** [End].

☛ **Type** ,2)↵

This should produce a value of 1.097815

The results above show that for any 1 unit change in the value of Fbg i.e. 1mmol per litre, there will be an approximate increase in Vcf of 0.22% per second. If we require further information, it is easier to use the method below. Before using this method, delete the values calculated by Method 1:

🖱 **Paint** D3 and D4.

☛ **Press** [Del].

5.7.2 Method 2

Method 2 gives far greater detail including labels to indicate values of various statistics.

From the menu bar:

🖱 **Select** 'Tools'.

🖱 **Select** 'Data Analysis'.

A list of tools appears, shown in Fig. 5.17.

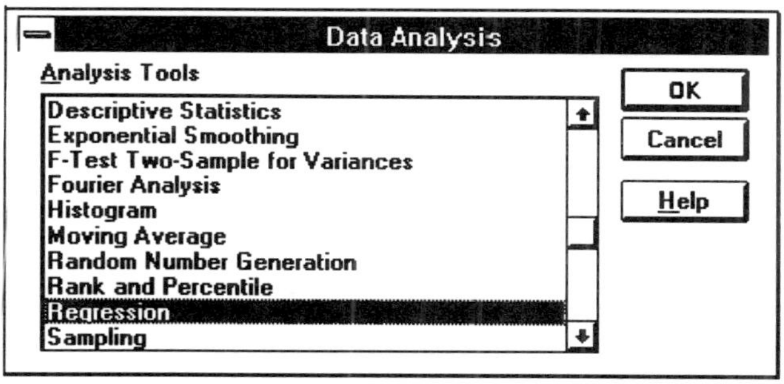

Fig 5.17 The Data Analysis tools.

> **Hint**: Wait while the file containing these tools is loaded. This may take some time!

Select 'Regression' from the box containing the analysis tools.

Click on OK.

A Regression dialog box will appear as shown in Fig. 5.18. We can now fill in the details to allow the regression to take place.

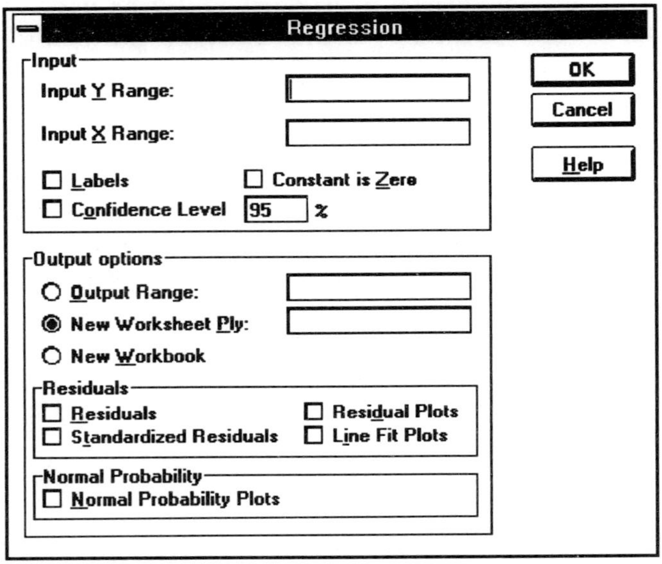

Fig. 5.18 Regression dialog box.

Click on 'Input Y Range'.

Type 'C3:C25' the values of the dependent variable.

Click on 'Input X Range'.

Type 'B3:B25' for the values of the independent variable.

Click on 'Output Range'.

Type D3.

Click on OK.

After a while the full results will be shown beginning at D3. The detailed statistics given by the system are beyond the scope of this text. Readers are recommended to read a suitable text such as that previously mentioned.

It is also possible to ask for values of the residuals (i.e. the differences between the actual and estimated values of Vcf for each value of Fbg) as well as a graph of the residuals plotted against the Fbg variable. This is useful in seeing whether there is a pattern in the residuals.

A pattern is usually indicative of the presence of one or more variables which have been left out of the analysis. The pattern will vary around a mean value of zero (as some residuals will be positive, some negative). Additionally we can ask for a line plot – a graph which shows the estimated values of Vcf against the actual values of Vcf. This again can often show patterns indicating the effect of other variables not included in the analysis. Fig. 5.19 illustrates the graph in the standard form produced by Excel's regression function.

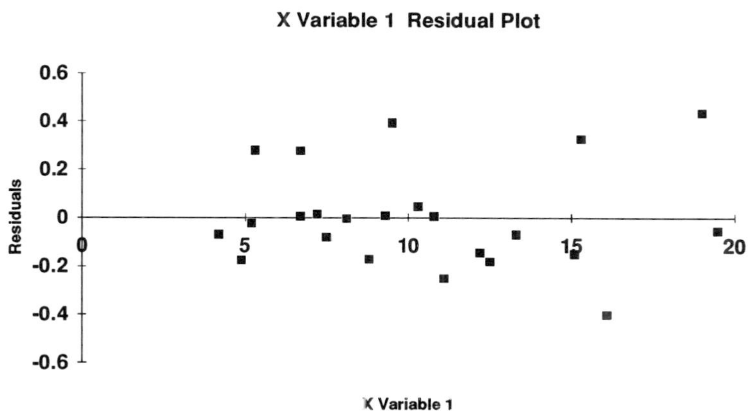

Fig. 5.19 Residual scatter plot.

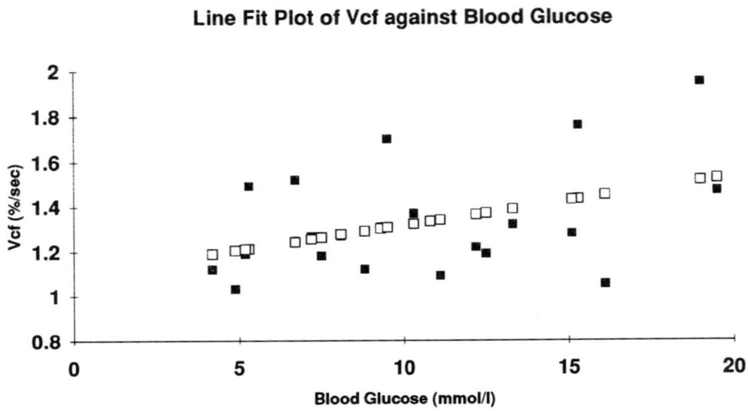

Fig. 5.20 Line fit plot of Vcf against blood glucose.

The titles can be amended to indicate the variables used in the analysis in the usual way as if it were a graph you produced yourself. The graph shown in Fig 5.20 has been amended in this way. The completed sheet produced by this process is stored as 'Glucose1.xls' and the results, which correspond to a line of best fit of

$$y = 0.022x + 1.09$$

are illustrated in Fig. 5.21. Note that this tallies with the earlier result obtained using the LINEST function.

> **Hint**: Some of the figures in Fig. 5.21 are shown to 2 decimal places to fit the results on one page.

	D	E	F	G	H	I
1						
2						
3	SUMMARY OUTPUT					
4						
5	*Regression Statistics*					
6	Multiple R	0.416755				
7	R Square	0.173684				
8	Adjusted R Square	0.134336				
9	Standard Error	0.216696				
10	Observations	23				
11						
12	ANOVA					
13		*df*	*SS*	*MS*	*F*	*Significance F*
14	Regression	1	0.207269	0.207269	4.414018	0.047896
15	Residual	21	0.986096	0.046957		
16	Total	22	1.193365			
17						

	D	E	F	G	H	I	J	K	L
18		*Coefficients*	*Standard Error*	*t Stat*	*P-value*	*Lower 95%*	*Upper 95%*	*Lower 95.000%*	*Upper 95.000%*
19	Intercept	1.09	0.11	9.34	6.26E-09	0.85	1.34	0.85	1.34
20	X Variable 1	0.021963	0.01	2.10	0.04	2E-04	0.04	2E-04	0.04
21									

Fig. 5.21 The regression results.

Many other statistical functions are provided in the analysis tool pack and some of them are listed in Table 5.4.

Table 5.4 The analysis tools.

Functions available within the analysis tool pack
Anova: single-factor
Anova: two-factor with replication
Anova: two-factor without replication
Correlation
Covariance
Descriptive statistics
Exponential smoothing
F-test: two-sample for variances
t-test: two-sample assuming equal variances
t-test: two-sample assuming unequal variances
t-test: paired two-sample for means
z-test: two-sample for means
Histogram
Moving average
Random number generation
Rank and percentile
Regression

6

Managing income and resources

6.1 CHAPTER SUMMARY

This chapter illustrates further aspects of managing income and resources through two examples. In the first example, you are given the job of drawing up a staffing rota for the practice. You need to minimize costs whilst ensuring adequate coverage at all times. You must also work within the constraints of the working conditions laid down by the agreements made with staff over existing working practices.

In the second, the practice is concerned with the use of resources and the match to doctor and patients in different age ranges. The spreadsheet is used to analyze the income from capitation by doctor and age range.

The issues covered in this chapter include:

- producing an optimal solution for a constrained problem;
- automating the solution;
- analyzing multidimensional data.

The following Excel features are included:

- the 'what if' problem solver;
- the use of macros for function and application automation;
- the pivot table facility.

6.2 MANAGING THE STAFFING BUDGET

Managing resources effectively is important because budgets are always finite. One of the most significant resources in terms of contribution and cost is the staff. Our example shows the 'what-if' feature of Excel can be used to optimize staffing arrangements within a large practice.

The scenario

A large practice is trying to establish how many reception staff are required to run the surgeries effectively. The staffing arrangements are subject to the following constraints:

- There are eleven sessions to be staffed, morning and evening, Monday to Friday and Saturday morning.
- No member of staff should be required to work more than 3 evening sessions.
- Each member of staff is entitled to two days off which may be taken continuously, in addition to Sunday.
- Each staff-session costs the practice £25.00
- Each session has its own staffing demand indicated by Table 6.1.

The aim is to provide a staffing rota that meets all the criteria set at the minimum cost. This problem has been set up for us in the example 'staffing.xls'. The sheet is illustrated in Fig. 6.1.

In order to see how the example works,

🖱 **Open** 'staffing.xls' .

Table 6.1 Staffing requirements by session.

Session	*Staff required*
Monday, a.m.	8
Monday, p.m.	6
Tuesday, a.m.	6
Tuesday, p.m.	4
Wednesday, a.m.	6
Wednesday, p.m.	4
Thursday, a.m.	6
Thursday, p.m.	4
Friday, a.m.	8
Friday, p.m.	6
Saturday, a.m.	4

Example : Reception Staff Scheduling for a large health centre.

For employees working eight sessions with four consecutive sessions off and not more than three evening sessions, find the schedule which meets demand from attendance levels while minimizing payroll costs.

Sch.	*Days off*	*Staff*	*Mon a.m.*	*Mon p.m.*	*Tue a.m.*	*Tues p.m.*	*Wed a.m.*	*Wed p.m.*	*Thurs a.m.*	*Thurs p.m.*	*Fri a.m.*	*Fri p.m.*	*Sat a.m.*
A	*Monday, Tuesday*	3	0	0	0	0	1	1	1	1	1	1	1
B	*Tuesday, Wed.*	3	1	1	0	0	0	0	1	1	1	1	1
C	*Wed., Thursday*	3	1	1	1	1	0	0	0	0	1	1	1
D	*Thursday, Friday*	3	1	1	1	1	1	1	0	0	0	0	1
E	*Friday, Saturday*	3	1	1	1	1	1	1	1	0	0	0	0
	Schedule Totals:	15	12	12	9	9	9	9	9	6	9	9	12
	Total Demand:		8	6	6	4	6	4	6	4	8	6	4

Cost/Employee/Session	***£25.00***	***Payroll/Week:***	**£2625.00**
Cost/Employee/Week:	***£175.00***		

Fig. 6.1 The worksheet 'staffing.xls'.

The data is divided into three sections. Rows 7-13 represent the staffing schedules. Each schedule allows the required two days off and does not require the staff to work more than three evening sessions. Attendance is shown by a 1. To start the analysis we suggest numbers of staff to put into each rota. The numbers should be large enough to ensure minimum cover is exceeded. In the absence of other data, each rota is set to the same size (3). These values are found in cells C9 to C13. These are the values that will be changed by the analysis.

Row 16 contains the staffing levels that the system calculates from these initial values. Row 18 contains the minimum staffing levels calculated from patient attendance patterns. At all times the values in Row 16 must exceed the values in Row 18.

In Rows 20 & 21, the actual cost is worked out by multiplying the cost of each member of staff by the number of staff required:

Cost per staff member per session	= £25
Cost per staff member per week	= £25 * 7 = £175
Total cost	= £175 * Number of staff

The aim of the analysis is to find the minimum value of the total payroll cost subject to the constraints already mentioned.

To carry out the analysis:

🖰 **Select** 'Tools'.

🖰 **Select** 'Solver'.

A dialog box appears to allow us to enter the parameters for the analysis. There are three parameters to be set:

1. The cell to be optimized containing a single output value.
2. The cells to be changed containing the input data.
3. The constraints upon optimization.

These values are entered into the respective boxes in our dialog box. The target value is contained in $J$20. This is the total staffing cost. This is to be minimized by changing $C$9:$C$13 subject to the three constraints shown below:

a) $C9:$C13= integer;

b) $C9:$C13>= 0;

c) $D$16:$N$16>=$DS18:$N$18.

Constraint a) says that the values in C9 to C13 must be whole numbers. Constraint b) says they must be positive. Constraint c) says that the values in the row D16 to N16 must be greater than the minimum requirements stored in cells D18 to N18.To implement this:

- **Click** in [box] next to 'Set Target Cell'.
- **Type** $J$20.
- **Select** Min.
- **Click** in [box] below 'By changing'.
- **Type** $C9:$C13.
- **Click** on [Add...].

The following dialog box appears:

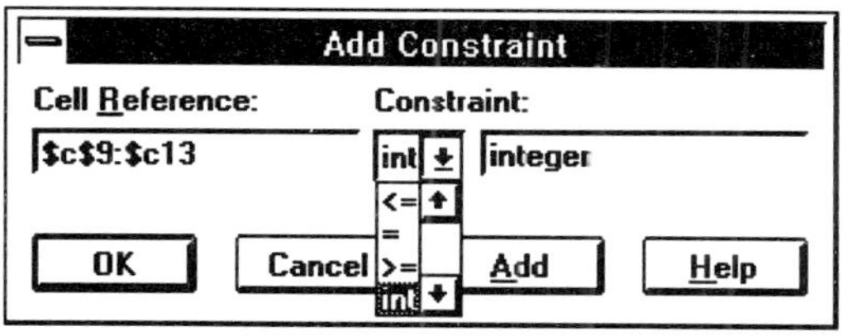

Fig. 6.2 The Add Constraint dialog box.

- **Type** $C9:$C13.
- **Click** on [↓]

From the drop down list,

- **Select** 'int'.
- **Click** on [Add...].
- **Type** $C9:$C13.
- **Click** on [↓]

From the drop down list,

Select >=.

Type 0 in the 'Constraint' box.

Click on Add....

Type $D$16:$N$16.

Click on ▼

From the drop down list,

Select >=.

Type $D$18:$N$18 in the 'Constraint' box..

Click on OK.

The finished dialog box should look like Fig. 6.3.

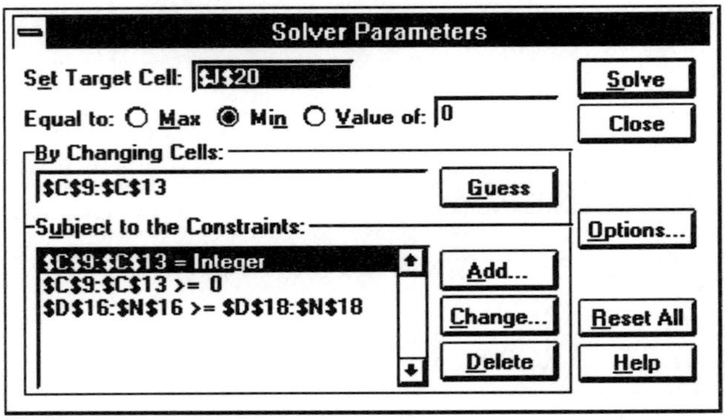

Fig. 6.3 The Solver Parameters dialog box.

Click on Solve.

The system sends messages to the status bar at the bottom of the screen informing you of what is happening. Once complete, another dialog box appears, asking whether any reports are required:

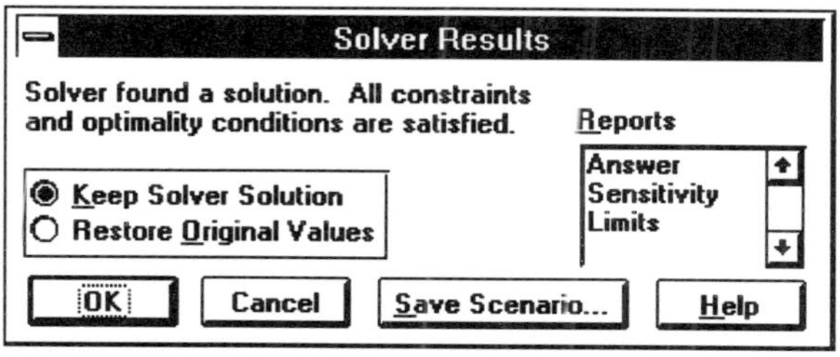

Fig. 6.4 Solver results dialog box.

Select 'Answer' from reports.

Click on OK.

The result is a full description of the analysis. First, let's look at the staffing sheet. The system has optimized the staffing levels and produced the ideal rotas:

Example : Reception Staff Scheduling for a large health centre.

For employees working eight sessions with four consecutive sessions off and not more than three evening sessions, find the schedule which meets demand from attendance levels while minimizing payroll costs.

Sch.	*Days off*	*Staff*	*Mon a.m.*	*Mon p.m.*	*Tue a.m.*	*Tues p.m.*	*Wed a.m.*	*Wed p.m.*	*Thurs a.m.*	*Thurs p.m.*	*Fri a.m.*	*Fri p.m.*	*Sat a.m.*
A	*Monday, Tuesday*	3	0	0	0	0	1	1	1	1	1	1	1
B	*Tuesday, Wed.*	1	1	1	0	0	0	0	1	1	1	1	1
C	*Wed., Thursday*	4	1	1	1	1	0	0	0	0	1	1	1
D	*Thursday, Friday*	0	1	1	1	1	1	1	0	0	0	0	1
E	*Friday, Saturday*	3	1	1	1	1	1	1	1	0	0	0	0
	Schedule Totals:	11	8	8	7	7	6	6	7	4	8	8	8
	Total Demand:		8	6	6	4	6	4	6	4	8	6	4
Cost/Employee/Session		***£25.00***					***Payroll/Week:***		**£1,925.00**				
Cost/Employee/Week:		***£175.00***											

Fig. 6.5 The optimized rota.

The minimum cost is found to be £1 925. This represents a saving of £700 on our initial estimate. For full details of the calculation, we may refer to the answer report. It may be found on a separate sheet labelled 'Answer Report 1'.

Click on Answer Report 1.

The report is shown in Fig. 6.6:

Microsoft Excel 5.0 Answer Report
Worksheet: [STAFFING.XLS]STAFFING
Report Created: 7/5/94
14:09

Target Cell (Min)

Cell	Name	Original Value	Final Value
$J$20	Payroll/Week: a.m.	£2625.00	£1925.00

Adjustable Cells

Cell	Name	Original Value	Final Value
$C$9	Monday, Tuesday Staff	3	3
$C$10	Tuesday, Wed. Staff	3	1
$C$11	Wed., Thursday Staff	3	4
$C$12	Thursday, Friday Staff	3	0
$C$13	Friday, Saturday Staff	3	3

Constraints

Cell	Name	Cell Value	Formula	Status	Slack
$D$16	Schedule Totals: a.m.	8	$D$16>=$D$18	Binding	0
$E$16	Schedule Totals: p.m.	8	$E$16>=$E$18	Not Binding	2
$F$16	Schedule Totals: a.m.	7	$F$16>=$F$18	Not Binding	1
$G$16	Schedule Totals: p.m.	7	$G$16>=$G$18	Not Binding	3
$H$16	Schedule Totals: a.m.	6	$H$16>=$H$18	Binding	0
$I$16	Schedule Totals: p.m.	6	$I$16>=$I$18	Not Binding	2
$J$16	Schedule Totals: a.m.	7	$J$16>=$J$18	Not Binding	1
$K$16	Schedule Totals: p.m.	4	$K$16>=$K$18	Binding	0
$L$16	Schedule Totals: a.m.	8	$L$16>=$L$18	Binding	0
$M$16	Schedule Totals: p.m.	8	$M$16>=$M$18	Not Binding	2
$C$9	Monday, Tuesday Staff	3	$C$9=integer	Binding	0
$C$10	Tuesday, Wed. Staff	1	$C$10=integer	Binding	0
$C$11	Wed., Thursday Staff	4	$C$11=integer	Binding	0
$C$12	Thursday, Friday Staff	0	$C$12=integer	Binding	0
$C$13	Friday, Saturday Staff	3	$C$13=integer	Binding	0
$C$9	Monday, Tuesday Staff	3	$C$9>=0	Not Binding	3
$C$10	Tuesday, Wed. Staff	1	$C$10>=0	Not Binding	1
$C$11	Wed., Thursday Staff	4	$C$11>=0	Not Binding	4
$C$12	Thursday, Friday Staff	0	$C$12>=0	Binding	0
$C$13	Friday, Saturday Staff	3	$C$13>=0	Not Binding	3

Fig 6.6 The answer report

Each constraint is listed as 'binding' or 'not binding'. A binding constraint is a critical limiting factor. If the constraint is listed as not binding then that variable does not limit the final solution. Thus in our problem, the key times when the staffing level is at the lowest permissible value are shown in Table 6.2:

Table 6.2 Critical times in optimized staff rota.

Critical times
Monday a.m.
Wednesday a.m.
Thursday p.m.
Friday a.m.

The slack column indicates spare capacity. Thus, a value of zero in the 'slack' column indicates a binding constraint. A value of greater than zero indicates that the constraint is not binding. The greater the value, the more slack is available with respect to that particular constraint.

We will return to this example for revision purposes at the end of the chapter. Save the solution as 'staff1.xls':

- **Select** 'File' from the menu bar.
- **Select** 'Save as'.
- **Type** 'staff1.xls'.
- **Click** on OK.

6.2.1 Automating procedures within Excel

The process of producing graphs in the previous chapters is quite quick, but requires us to go through a considerable number of selections. It would be useful to be able to automate these stages and produce a graph with a single action. This may be achieved using a **command macro**. A macro is a collection of commands which may be implemented as a group.

We shall now construct a general purpose command macro to produce a 3-D column chart from any painted area. First, return to the original data sheet by selecting the tab at the bottom of the sheet. Next, we select the area to graphed:

- **Paint** cells D7 to N7.
- **Hold down** the [Ctrl] key and **paint** cells D18 to N18.

Now we are ready to define the command macro:

- **Select** 'Tools' from the menu.
- **Select** the 'Record Macro' option.
- **Select** 'Record New Macro'.

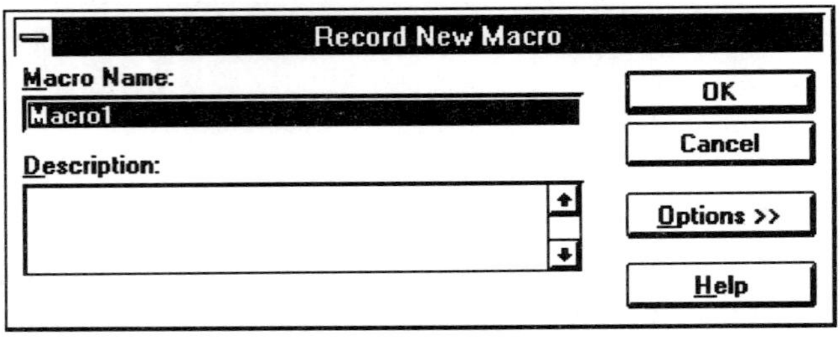

Fig. 6.7 The Record New Macro dialog box.

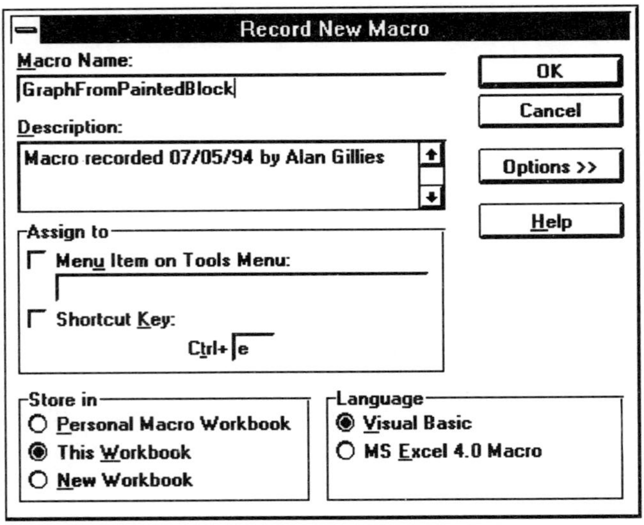

Fig. 6.8 Expanded Record New Macro dialog box.

Type GraphFromPaintedBlock.

Click on [Options >>].

The dialog box expands to offer a range of options, illustrated in Fig. 6.8.

The macro we are developing will produce a graph from any painted area, so it is a global macro and can be used with any spreadsheet. Therefore, we will include it in our personal macro workbook.

Select 'Personal Macro Workbook'.

Click on [OK].

> **Hint:** The personal macro workbook provides a repository for general purpose macros which you may wish to access from any Excel workbook. If a macro is specific to one workbook, it is better to store it on its own sheet within the workbook.

When the macro starts, a 'stop' button, as depicted below, will appear towards the top right corner of the screen. This may be used at any time to stop recording.

Now we enter the commands for the macro itself:

Select 'Insert' from the menu bar.

Select 'Chart'.

Select 'As new sheet'.

Right-click on the chart to access the short cut menu.

Select Chart type.

Select '3-D'.

Select '3-D Column'.

Click on [OK].

Click on the legend.

Press [Del].

Now stop recording the commands for the macro:

Click on 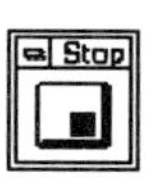

.

What should be on the screen is the chart shown in Fig. 6.9.

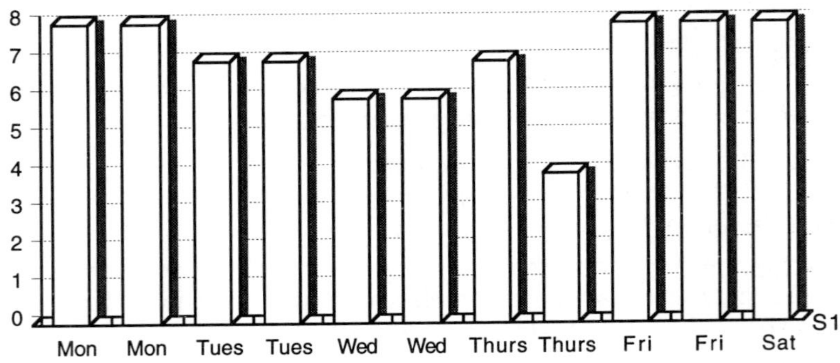

Fig. 6.9 Resulting chart.

We can add a title. The following procedure is the one to be used when chart details such as title have not been added at the time of original chart production.

- **Select** 'Insert' from the menu bar.
- **Select** 'Titles'.
- **Click** ☒ on Chart Title.
- **Click** on [OK].

The word 'Title' will now appear surrounded by small squares. Use the Backspace key (←)to remove the word 'Title', and replace with 'Staffing requirements for the practice'. Now repeat the process by using the macro to help plot the results of our analysis. First return to the staffing data sheet, then:

- **Paint** cells D7 to N7.
- ☛ **Hold down** the [Ctrl] key and **paint** cells D16 to N16.
- **Select** 'Tools'.
- **Select** 'Macro'.
- **Select** GraphFromPaintedBlock.

Click on ‘Run’.

The macro now produces a graph for the optimized data.
Now add a title to the new graph:

Select ‘Insert’ from the menu bar.

Select ‘Titles’.

Click ☒ on Chart Title.

Click on [OK].

To enter the actual text, as an alternative to the procedure above:

Click on the editing bar.

☛ **Type** Optimized staffing levels for the practice↵.

We can even start a macro from a button on one of the toolbars. The first stage in this operation is to put a suitable button on one of the toolbars:

Select ‘View’ from the menu bar.

Select ‘Toolbars’.

Click on ‘Customize’.

Select ‘Charting’ from the ‘Categories’ list.

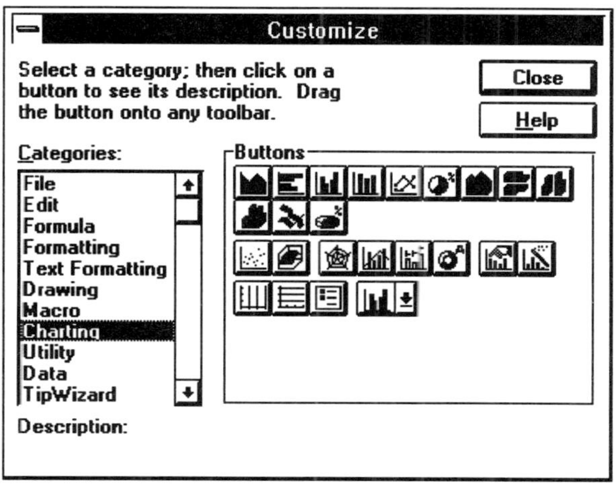

Fig. 6.10 Customize dialog box.

Fig. 6.10 shows the selection of buttons available in the Charting toolbar.

Click on  the 3D Chart.

Drag it up to the Standard toolbar at the top of the screen and release.

The 3-D Chart button should now be in position on the toolbar with a dotted edge. Currently the use of the 3D Chart button would cause the system to create a 3-D Chart only if a selected area were to be painted in but the operation of the button can be customized so that it runs the macro which has been created earlier.

Select 'Tools'.

Select 'Assign Macro'.

Select GraphFromPaintedBlock.

Click on [OK].

Click on [Close] in the Customize dialog box.

The Macro can now be run directly by pressing the button. This routine is especially useful if the same procedure is to be used over and over again using different data sets to produce graphs and charts. As an exercise, choose a data row from the staffing sheet, paint the cells then click on the new button installed in the toolbar.

So far we have produced a general purpose macro. Now we shall use a locally defined macro to enhance our sheet. First we need to do a little re-arranging to allow the system to produce a more complex graph for us. The re-arranged sheet is called 'Staff2.xls'.

We shall first create two buttons to give us access to local macros:

Click on , the Drawing Tool.

A drawing toolbar will appear.

Click on  to create a button.

When the icon is moved away from the Drawing Toolbar, a cross will appear.

Drag the mouse to outline the button at the bottom of the screen.

The words 'Button 1' will appear in the button. After a few seconds the 'Assign Macro' dialog box will appear.

Click on 'Record'.

Type a name in the macro name box.

Click on 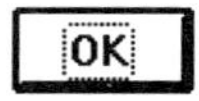.

A Stop Record button will appear after a few seconds.

Select 'Tools'.

Select 'Solver'.

The parameters have not changed, so we may

Click on 'Solve'.

When the analysis is complete:

Click on 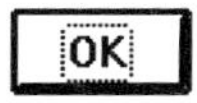 without selecting any reports.

Click on 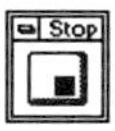, the Stop Record button.

Hold down the [Ctrl] button.

Click on the button labelled 'Button 1'.

Replace 'Button 1' with 'Optimize' (by typing at the keyboard).

> **Health Warning**: Do not press return after completing the text. This takes you to the next line in the button text. Instead, complete by clicking on another portion of the sheet.

Now we can add another button to show the results graphically:

Click  the Drawing Tool, if it is not already showing.

The drawing toolbar will appear.

Click on  to create a button.

Drag the mouse to outline the button at the bottom of the screen.

The words 'Button 2' will appear in the button. After a few seconds the 'Assign Macro' dialog box will appear:

Click on 'Record'.

- **Type** a name for the macro in the Macro dialog box.
- **Click** on OK.

A Stop Record button will now appear.

- Paint cells D7 to N7.

> **Hint**: If the drawing tool bar is in the way, close it down by:
>
> - **Double-click** on its control box.

- **Hold down** the [Ctrl] key and **paint** cells D16 to N16.
- **Hold down** the [Ctrl] key and **paint** cells D18 to N18.
- **Click** on the Chart Wizard.
- **Drag** the cursor to create a graph within the sheet.
- **Click** on the 3-D column graph New option.
- **Click** on Next >.
- **Click** on 'Format 1'.
- **Click** on Next > twice to move to Step 5 in chart production.
- **Type** in the words 'Optimized staffing levels compared with minimum requirements' as a title. Make any other appropriate changes to the graph.
- **Click** on Finish.
- **Select** Stop, the Stop Record button.
- **Hold** down the [Ctrl] button and **click** on Button 2.
- **Replace** with 'Show Results' (by typing at the keyboard).

Show Results

To obtain the image shown here, press return after the word 'Show' and then type in the word 'Results'. Then click on another portion of the sheet to finish. If you have not drawn the button large enough not all the text will be shown. The button can be re-sized according to need by firstly holding down the [Ctrl] key and clicking on the button. The button will then be outlined. By pointing at a corner of the button the diagonal re-sizing icon will appear allowing you to drag the button into the appropriate shape. Now we have a customized application, we can test different scenarios with our model. First we shall test the results by returning the data to our original estimates:

- **Click** on C9.
- **Type** 3.
- **Autofill** across from C9 to C13.

Save this sheet as 'Staff3.xls' before you go any further and then delete the graph sheet. To delete the graph sheet, first select it by its tab at the bottom of the sheet, then

- **Select** 'Edit' from the menu bar.
- **Select** 'Delete sheet'.
- **Click** on the 'Optimize' button. A hand will appear.
- Choose your report at the dialog box or **click** on [OK] to produce none.
- **Click** on 'Show Results' to display the result as a 3-D column chart.

Now imagine the surgery gets busier. Staffing demand rises. Enter these new demand figures into cells D16 to N16:

8	6	8	4	8	4	8	4	8	8	4

As workload has risen we should raise our 'guesstimates' to 4:

Set C9 to C13 equal to 4.

- **Click** on the 'Optimize' button.
- Choose your report at the dialog box or **click** on [OK] to produce none.
- **Click** on 'Show Results' to display the result as a 3-D column chart.

6.3 ANALYZING CAPITATION INCOME

Basic income for general practice is derived from capitation. The capitation fee is paid per patient and varies according to the age of the patient:

Table 6.3 Capitation fees (1993).

Patient's age	*Capitation fee*
under 65	£14.30
65-74	£18.85
75 and over	£36.45

In order to manage resources properly it is useful to calculate the capitation income from each age group and by doctor. This can be done using the pivot table facility in Excel. The workbook, 'capita.xls' contains information about patients registered in each age band with three doctors in a practice: Drs Brown, Green and White. The data is broken down into the appropriate age bands.

- **Open** capita.xls.
- **Click** on OK.
- **Click** on H1.
- **Type** Q1↵.
- **Autofill** across from H1 to K1.
- **Paint** H2 to K10.
- **Select** 'Format' from the menu bar.
- **Select** 'Cells'.
- **Select** the currency category.
- **Select** £#.##0;-£#.##0.

Click on OK.

Click on H2.

Type =$G2*C2.

Autofill across from H2 to K2.

Autofill the cells H2 to K2 down to H10 to K10.

Select 'Data' from the menu bar.

Select 'Pivot Table'.

This brings the PivotTable Wizard onto the screen. This consists of four stages, illustrated in Fig. 6.11:

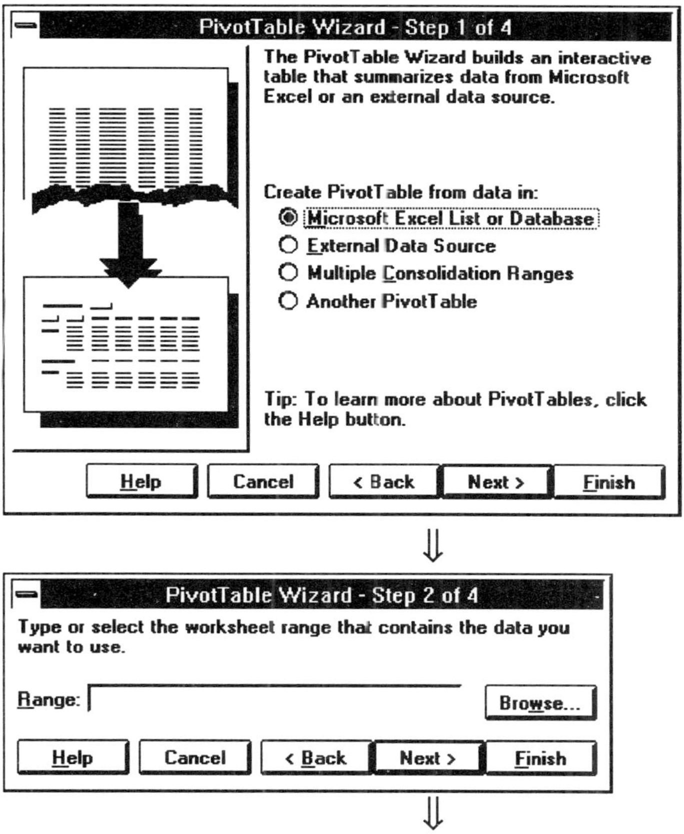

Fig. 6.11 The PivotTable Wizard.

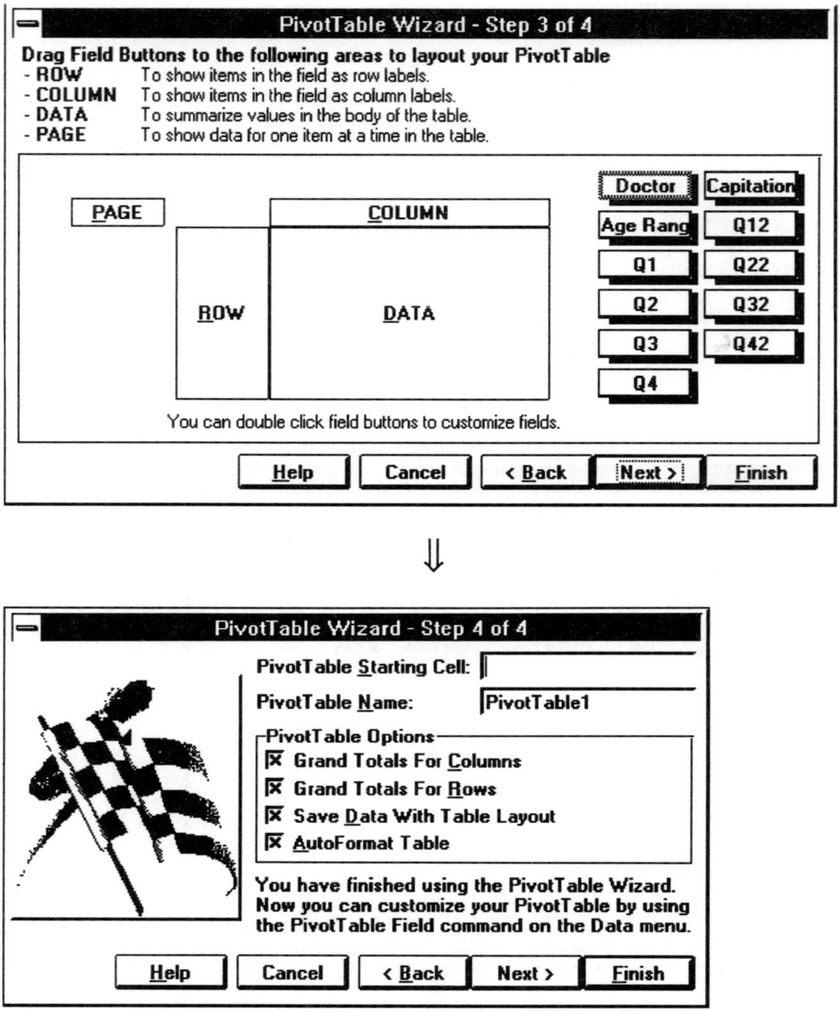

Fig. 6.11 The PivotTable Wizard (continued).

In step 1, we select the data source type. The default is an Excel list or database, so we simply

Click on [Next >].

In step 2, we select the data range:

☛ **Type** a1:k10↵.

> **Hint**: Pressing the ↵ key after typing the data range moves us automatically to step 3, omitting the need to click on **Next >**.

To set up the pivot table, drag the buttons from the right hand side of the step 3 dialog box shown in Fig. 6.12 onto the table:

- **Drag** Q12 onto DATA.
- **Drag** Q22 onto DATA.
- **Drag** Q32 onto DATA.
- **Drag** Q42 onto DATA.
- **Drag** Age Range onto ROW.
- **Drag** Doctor onto COLUMN.

The net effect is illustrated in Fig. 6.12.

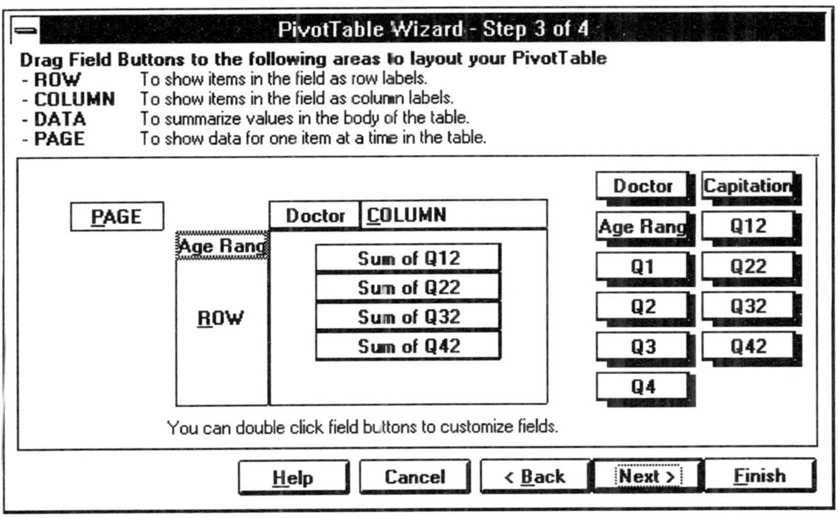

Fig. 6.12 PivotTable Wizard: completed step 3 dialog box.

- **Click** on **Next >**.

In the step 4 dialog box, the destination cell determines where Excel places the resulting table. In this case, we shall place the result in a separate sheet in the same workbook:

- **Type** sheet2!a1↵.

	A	B	C	D	E	F
1			Doctor			
2	Age Range	Data	Brown	Green	White	Grand Total
3	-65	Sum of Q12	16530.8	10939.5	22408.1	49878.4
4		Sum of Q22	17088.5	10553.4	22222.2	49864.1
5		Sum of Q32	17231.5	10825.1	22737	50793.6
6		Sum of Q42	17002.7	10882.3	23008.7	50893.7
7	65-74	Sum of Q12	4354.35	3524.95	4561.7	12441
8		Sum of Q22	4524	3468.4	4712.5	12704.9
9		Sum of Q32	4524	3524.95	4806.75	12855.7
10		Sum of Q42	4561.7	3656.9	4844.45	13063.05
11	74+	Sum of Q12	3572.1	2660.85	4483.35	10716.3
12		Sum of Q22	3535.65	2733.75	4483.35	10752.75
13		Sum of Q32	3572.1	2770.2	4374	10716.3
14		Sum of Q42	3499.2	2806.65	4264.65	10570.5
15	Total Sum of Q12		24457.3	17125.3	31453.15	73035.7
16	Total Sum of Q22		25148.2	16755.6	31418.05	73321.75
17	Total Sum of Q32		25327.6	17120.3	31917.75	74365.6
18	Total Sum of Q42		25063.6	17345.9	32117.8	74527.25

Fig. 6.13 Resulting pivot table in sheet2.

The pivot table is placed in the top left hand corner of sheet2, and should look like the result illustrated in Fig. 6.13. The resulting pivot table in sheet2 should be reformatted as currency format:

- **Paint** C3 to F18.
- **Select** 'Format' from the menu bar.
- **Select** 'Cells'.
- **Select** 'Number'.
- **Select** the currency category.
- **Select** £#.##0;-£#.##0.
- **Click** on OK.

We can now customize the pivot table to focus on particular aspects of interest:

- **Click** on Sheet1.
- **Paint** A1 to K10.
- **Select** 'Data' from the menu bar.

Select 'Pivot Table'.

Because we have pre-selected the data for analysis (Sheet1, A1 to K10), the PivotTable Wizard proceeds to Step 3:

Drag Q12 onto the table.

Drag Age Range onto ROW.

Drag Doctor onto COLUMN.

Now we can tailor the data from the first quarter to our specific requirements:

Double-click on Sum of Q12.

The following dialog box appears (Fig. 6.14):

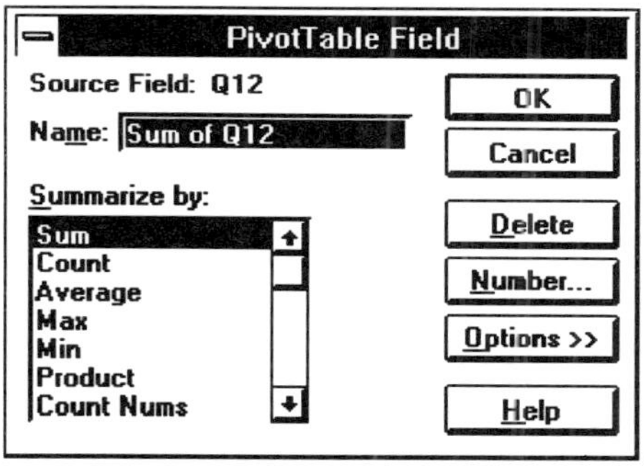

Fig. 6.14 PivotTable Field dialog box.

Click on Options >>.

Select '% of row' from the drop down list in the 'Show Data As' box.

Click on OK.

Click on Next >.

Type sheet3!a1↵ for the starting cell.

The resulting table shows the contribution to total capitation income sub-divided by doctor, for each age band and their overall contribution.

This may be further illustrated by plotting a pie chart next to the data table.

Paint B2 to D2.

Hold down the [Ctrl] key and **Paint** B6 to D6.

Click on [chart icon].

Drag the [chart cursor] cursor to enclose an area overlying the cells G2 to J12.

Click on [Next >].

Click on 'Pie'.

Click on [Next >].

Click on [Next >].

Click on [Next >].

Type Capitation by doctor↵.

and a pie chart will appear on the worksheet. We can alternatively break our data down by age range.

Click on \Sheet1/.

Paint A1 to K10.

Select 'Data' from the menu bar.

Select 'Pivot Table'.

Double-click on Sum of Q12.

Click on [Options >>].

Select '% of column' from the drop down list in the 'Show Data As' box.

Click on [OK].

Click on [Next >].

Type sheet3!a12↵.

The completed sheet3 is shown in Fig. 6.15.

The pivot table technique can be used to analyze data, not just from Excel workbooks, but also from other data sources. External data formats supported include Dbase, Access, Foxpro and Oracle.

	A	B	C	D	E
1	Sum of Q12	Doctor			
2	Age Range	Brown	Green	White	Grand Total
3	-65	33.14%	21.93%	44.93%	100.00%
4	65-74	35.00%	28.33%	36.67%	100.00%
5	74+	33.33%	24.83%	41.84%	100.00%
6	Grand Total	33.49%	23.45%	43.07%	100.00%
7					
8					
9					
10					
11					
12	Sum of Q12	Doctor			
13	Age Range	Brown	Green	White	Grand Total
14	-65	67.59%	63.88%	71.24%	68.29%
15	65-74	17.80%	20.58%	14.50%	17.03%
16	74+	14.61%	15.54%	14.25%	14.67%
17	Grand Total	100.00%	100.00%	100.00%	100.00%

Fig. 6.15 Resulting pivot table in sheet3.

6.4 REVISION EXERCISES

6.4.1 The Solver staffing example

1. Now return to the chart and display the optimum staffing levels for the eleven sessions: choose whatever graphical format you think is appropriate.

2. Enhance the graph by showing the minimum required levels on the same axes.

3. Now re-load the original staffing.xls sheet. Change the constraints so that the minimum number of staff on any one schedule is 1 instead of zero. What does this tell you ?

6.4.2 The PivotTable example

1. Construct tables corresponding to that shown in Fig. 6.15 for quarters 2,3 and 4.

2. Draw a stacked column chart showing the capitation income for each doctor, broken down by age range.

7

Medical audit

7.1 CHAPTER SUMMARY

Medical audit is a major and growing part of the activity of the National Health Service in the UK. This chapter will show how Excel can be used as an analysis tool within the medical audit process. It will use as an example an audit considering the quality of care received by patients attending an outpatient orthopaedic clinic.

This chapter covers:

- constructing a frequency distribution table;
- constructing a frequency distribution chart;
- using a chi-squared test to evaluate relationships between variables;
- revision exercises of techniques from the rest of the book.

The following features of Excel are covered:

- compound statements;
- combining logical and numerical formulae;
- managing multiple worksheets within a workbook;
- the CHITEST() function.

7.2 THE AUDIT

The outpatient orthopaedic clinic at Knapford General Hospital is extremely busy. There have been reports of patients experiencing delays before seeing the doctor. This audit has been established to investigate the extent of the problem.

Patients attending the clinic during the first six months of 1992 were asked to fill in a simple questionnaire. The questionnaire was given out to patients on arrival at the clinic. The patients were given the opportunity to return the form at the end of the visit. During this time, 1054 patients visited the clinic. Of these, 762 returned the forms, of which 733 were suitable for analysis.

The survey focused upon the patients' experiences before entering the consulting room. The audit asked the patients for the length of time between their appointment time and the actual time that they got to see the doctor. The respondents were also asked for their perceptions of the experience.

The survey targeted children particularly and their parents. Thus child patients are identified and their parents' responses analyzed separately. 257 of the 762 patients in the survey were in this category.

The aim of the audit is:

> 'to investigate the patients' view of care in an outpatient clinic.'

If we pursue this further, then we may define a specific set of objectives which arise from this overall aim, i.e. to determine

1. waiting times between referral and appointment;
2. waiting times within the clinic to see a doctor;
3. patient satisfaction with waiting times;
4. patient satisfaction with the waiting environment;
5. the level of experience of the doctor who saw the patients.

Each of these objectives then defines the data and analysis requirements of the audit.

7.2.1 The data

To meet objective 1, it is necessary to collect two pieces of data for each patient, the date of a request for an appointment and the date of the actual appointment. These are date fields and may be gathered from patient records.

The analysis method is to establish the time between the two dates as a number of days (t) and to consider performance in terms of t. To gather a rounded picture of t, the following information is required: the mean value of t, the dispersion measured as the standard deviation of t, and a column chart of the distribution of t.

Similarly, in order to establish waiting times in the clinic itself, it is necessary to monitor time of appointment and the actual time to see the doctor. This cannot be carried out retrospectively from records as it is not usual to record the time the patient was actually seen. This data would have to be recorded separately.

The data could be gathered from patients, since a patient questionnaire is required to address objective 3. To satisfy objective 3, it would be necessary to elicit patient views from a question such as the first one shown in Table 7.1.

Table 7.1 Sample question for patient questionnaire

How satisfied were you with the length of time you had to wait to see a doctor at the clinic?	
1. Very satisfied	[ ]
2. Quite satisfied	[ ]
3. No strong feelings	[ ]
4. Quite dissatisfied	[ ]
5. Very dissatisfied	[ ]
How did you feel about the waiting area at the clinic?	
1. Very satisfied	[ ]
2. Quite satisfied	[ ]
3. No strong feelings	[ ]
4. Quite dissatisfied	[ ]
5. Very dissatisfied	[ ]

This could be recorded as a numerical satisfaction measure (n_S) ranging from 1 to 5. In order to meet objective 4, a similar approach could be adopted, based around a question such as the second illustrated in Table 7.1.

In order to meet objective 5, it is necessary to record the status of the doctor, either as consultant (C), or registrar (R) or senior house officer (S). This leads to the set of data and analysis requirements summarized in Table 7.2, where, for example, ΣC refers to the number of patients seen by a consultant.

Table 7.2 Data requirements associated with each objective

	Objective 1	*Objective 2*	*Objective 3*	*Objective 4*	*Objective 5*
Data	requested date, app'tment date	app'tment time time seen	satisfaction measure	satisfaction measure	doctor status
Fields	$[D_{req}]$,$[D_{app}]$	$[T_{req}]$, $[T_{app}]$	numerical $n_S >= -2$ $n_S <= 2$	numerical $n_S >= -2$ $n_S <= 2$	alpha-numeric 'C','R','S'
Source	patient records	patient records, 'live' data	'live' data	'live' data	patient or clinic records
Analysis	$t=[D_{req}]-[D_{app}]$ t_{mean}, t_{stdev} histogram of t	$\Delta T=[T_{req}]-[T_{app}]$ ΔT_{mean}, ΔT_{stdev} histogram of ΔT	n_S mean. n_S stdev. histogram of n_S	n_S mean. n_S stdev. histogram of n_S	ΣC, ΣR, ΣS.

It is also necessary to decide whether there is any subsidiary data required to break down the groups further. For example, the audit introduction identifies child patients as a priority group within the study. Thus, it is necessary to include a data field for a child patient, stored as a 'Yes/No' field, allowing the overall results to be broken down in this way.

7.2.2 The analysis

The data collected by the audit is stored in the sheet 'audit.xls'.

Open audit.xls.

The first twenty records from a total of 733 in the dataset are shown in Fig. 7.1:

	A	B	C	D	E	F	G	H
1	PATIENT	REQUEST	APPTMENT	TIMEDUE	TIMESEEN	SATIS1	SATIS2	CHILD
2	1	27-Oct-91	30-Jan-92	1400	1500	2	1	Y
3	2	17-Nov-91	24-Feb-92	1430	1441	5	3	N
4	3	16-May-92	08-Jun-92	1530	1619	5	1	N
5	4	26-Jan-92	20-Mar-92	1530	1643	4	5	N
6	5	05-Nov-91	17-Feb-92	1530	1543	5	2	N
7	6	29-Nov-91	10-Feb-92	1430	1458	5	2	Y
8	7	02-Jan-92	28-Jan-92	1445	1522	5	1	N
9	8	10-Mar-92	09-Apr-92	1445	1448	5	1	N
10	9	28-Jan-92	25-Apr-92	1515	1628	5	2	N
11	10	30-Jan-92	15-Apr-92	1400	1522	5	5	N
12	11	05-Mar-92	16-Apr-92	1430	1447	5	5	N
13	12	15-Nov-91	17-Jan-92	1515	1533	5	4	N
14	13	01-Dec-91	02-Mar-92	1430	1458	5	4	Y
15	14	25-Nov-91	11-Mar-92	1530	1637	3	3	Y
16	15	25-Nov-91	05-Jan-92	1400	1519	2	5	N
17	16	03-Jun-92	27-Jun-92	1400	1508	3	2	Y
18	17	03-Nov-91	09-Jan-92	1400	1538	4	1	N
19	18	18-Apr-92	01-Jun-92	1500	1616	3	5	N
20	19	24-Dec-91	30-Mar-92	1415	1418	5	4	N
21	20	25-Jan-92	31-Mar-92	1415	1458	5	5	N

Fig. 7.1 The first twenty records from the audit

The first piece of analysis we shall carry out is a frequency table for the two satisfaction ratings. To do this we shall first create a new worksheet within the work book:

Select 'Insert' from the menu bar.

Select 'Worksheet' option.

Next we shall build our frequency table using compound statements. First we will enter the labels:

Click on A1.

☛ **Type** How satisfied were you with the length of time you had to wait to see a doctor at the clinic?↵.

🖱 **Click** on A2.

☛ **Type** Very satisfied ↵.

🖱 **Click** on A3.

☛ **Type** Quite satisfied ↵.

🖱 **Click** on A4.

☛ **Type** No strong feelings↵.

🖱 **Click** on A5.

☛ **Type** Quite dissatisfied ↵.

🖱 **Click** on A6.

☛ **Type** Very dissatisfied ↵.

Now we shall use a compound statement to calculate the number of patients who rated their satisfaction with the waiting time as '1. Very satisfied':

🖱 **Click** on B2.

Type =SUM(IF(Sheet1!F$2:F$734=1,1,0)) (Do not press ↵!).

☛ Press [Ctrl] and [⇧] and ↵ simultaneously to tell Excel that this is a compound statement.

> **Hint:** We have encountered compond statements before in Chapter Four: please refer back if you are unsure.

The answer should be 8.

Now we shall copy and edit the formula:

🖱 **Autofill** down from B2 to B6.

🖱 **Double-click** on B3 after the =1 and before the comma.

☛ **Press** ← .

☛ **Type** 2.

☛ **Press** [Ctrl] and [⇧] and ↵ simultaneously.

🖱 **Double-click** on B4 after the =1 and before the comma.

☛ **Press** ← .

☛ **Type** 3.

☛ **Press** [Ctrl] and [⇧] and ↵ simultaneously.

🖱 **Double-click** on B5 after the =1 and before the comma.

☛ **Press** ← .

☛ **Type** 4.

☛ **Press** [Ctrl] and [⇧] and ↵ simultaneously.

🖱 **Double-click** on B6 after the =1 and before the comma.

☛ **Press** ← .

☛ **Type** 5.

☛ **Press** [Ctrl] and [⇧] and ↵ simultaneously.

The completed table should contain the following values:

Table 7.3 Frequency distribution table

How satisfied were you with the length of time you had to wait to see a doctor at the clinic?	
Very satisfied	8
Quite satisfied	62
No strong feelings	118
Quite dissatisfied	175
Very dissatisfied	370

The formulae required to produce these results are shown in Table 7.4.

Table 7.4 Formulae required for frequency distribution table

Row	*Label in column A*	*Formula in column B*
2	Very satisfied	=SUM(IF(SHEET1!F$2:F$734=1,1,0))
3	Quite satisfied	=SUM(IF(SHEET1!F$2:F$734=2,1,0))
4	No strong feelings	=SUM(IF(SHEET1!F$2:F$734=3,1,0))
5	Quite dissatisfied	=SUM(IF(SHEET1!F$2:F$734=4,1,0))
6	Very dissatisfied	=SUM(IF(SHEET1!F$2:F$734=5,1,0))

Now we can add a frequency distribution chart to our workbook.

Paint B2 to B6.

Select 'Insert' from the menu bar.

Select 'Chart'.

Select 'As New Sheet'.

The rest is up to you – this is all revision from earlier chapters. A suggested format is shown in Fig 7.2.

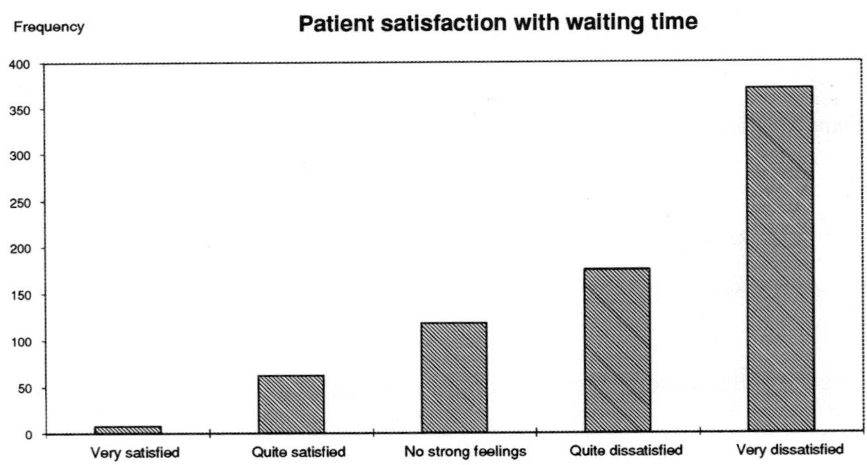

Fig. 7.2 Frequency distribution column chart.

Health warning: This is not a frequency histogram. True histograms are only accessible through the add-in analysis tool pack.

Now return to the sheet with the frequency table to add the frequency table for the second question. We shall copy the first table and then edit it to meet our requirements.

- **Paint** A2 to B6.
- **Click** on .
- **Click** on A9.
- **Click** on .
- **Press** [Esc] to remove outline marquee.
- **Click** on A8.
- **Type** How did you feel about the waiting area at the clinic?↵.
- **Paint** B9 to B13.
- **Select** 'Edit' from the menu bar.
- **Select** 'Replace' option.
- **Type** F$ ⇥ G$.

The dialog box should look like the one illustrated in Fig. 7.3.

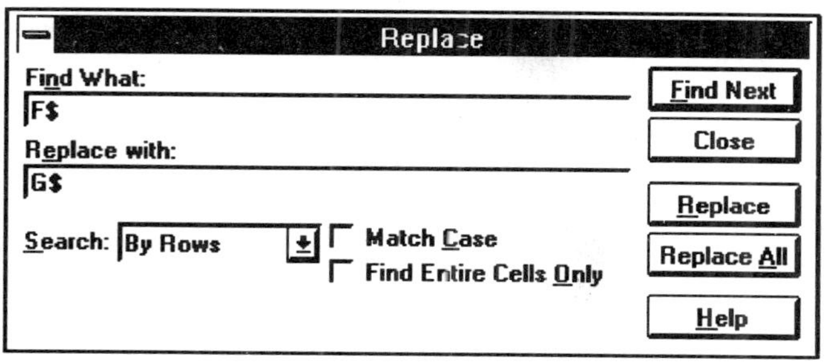

Fig. 7.3 The Replace dialog box

- **Press** Replace All to activate the replace option.

The resulting frequency distribution table looks like this:

Table 7.5 Frequency distribution table

How did you feel about the waiting area at the clinic?	
Very satisfied	165
Quite satisfied	137
No strong feelings	190
Quite dissatisfied	149
Very dissatisfied	92

Table 7.6 Formulae required for frequency distribution table

Row	*Label in column A*	*Formula in column B*
9	Very satisfied	=SUM(IF(SHEET1!G$2:G$734=1,1,0))
10	Quite satisfied	=SUM(IF(SHEET1!G$2:G$734=2,1,0))
11	No strong feelings	=SUM(IF(SHEET1!G$2:G$734=3,1,0))
12	Quite dissatisfied	=SUM(IF(SHEET1!G$2:G$734=4,1,0))
13	Very dissatisfied	=SUM(IF(SHEET1!G$2:G$734=5,1,0))

The formulae required to produce these results are shown in Table 7.6.

Now we may add a second column chart to our workbook to illustrate the results from this second question. This is left to the reader as an exercise. Remember to put the chart on a separate sheet. Our workbook will then contain four separate sheets. This illustrates how the workbook idea may be used to arrange data and resulting analysis in a logical manner.

Each audit investigation should have its own workbook, and within each, there may be many different sheets each concerned with a different analysis or chart. Once we have more than one sheet it is useful to give meaningful names to each sheet.

To name each sheet:

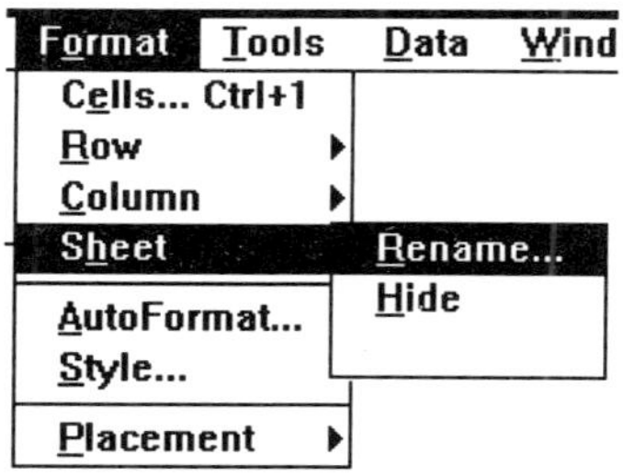

Fig 7.4 Renaming a sheet.

- **Select** 'Format' from the menu bar.
- **Select** 'Sheet'.
- **Select** 'Rename'.
- **Type** a suitable name for the sheet, see Table 7.7 below for suggestions.
- **Click** on OK.

Table 7.7 Suggested names for each sheet

Sheet	*Suggested names*
main sheet	Main data
sheet1	Freq dist
chart1	Freq chart1
chart2	Freq chart2

Repeat for each sheet. The names appear on the tabs at the bottom of the sheet:

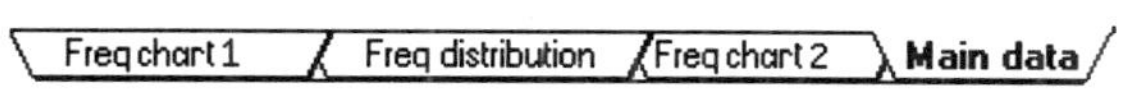

Fig 7.5 Names for sheets appear on tabs at the bottom.

We shall add a further sheet to investigate whether there is a relationship between the two responses. In other words, are people's impressions of the waitng room governed largely by the length of time they spend in them?

To do this, we shall use a chi-squared test.

First, we shall create a new worksheet:

🖱 **Select** 'Insert' from the menu bar.

🖱 **Select** 'Worksheet'.

Now add a name:

🖱 **Select** 'Format' from the menu bar.

🖱 **Select** 'Sheet'.

🖱 **Select** 'Rename'.

☛ **Type** Chi sqrd↵.

The chi-squared test is used to establish whether there is a relationship between two factors. We shall use it to establish whether there is a link between the satisfaction ratings for waiting time and the waiting area.

In order to carry out a chi-squared test we must define three things:

- a table of actual values;
- a null hypothesis;
- a table of expected values for the null hypothesis.

The table of actual values is constructed by cross-tabulating the two variables in this case, the satisfaction with the waiting time and the satisfaction with the waiting area:

	Waiting time						
Waiting		1	2	3	4	5	Total
area	1						
	2						A
	3						
	4						
	5						
	Total				B		C

Fig. 7.6 Cross-tabulated values for actual values table.

In Fig. 7.6, 1 is very satisfied, 2 is quite satisfied, 3 is no strong feelings, 4 is quite dissatisfied and 5 is very dissatisfied. A is the total number of responses quite satisfied with the waiting area, B is the total number of responses quite dissatisfied with the waiting time and C is the total sample.

Thus, the shaded cell in Fig. 7.6 contains the number of respondents who were quite satisfied with the waiting area and quite dissatisfied with the waiting time.

The null hypothesis states that there is no relationship between the factors. The chi squared probability gives us the probability that the null hypothesis is true. A probability close to one implies that the null hypothesis is true, and there is no relationship. A probability of close to zero implies that the null hypothesis is false and therefore there is a relationship.

We now calculate the table of values which we would expect if there was no relationship, that is, the null hypothesis is true. These values are calculated as follows:

$$\frac{\text{Row total x Column total}}{\text{Sample total}}$$

This represents the cross-section of a truly random sample. In terms of Fig. 7.6, the value in the shaded cell of the table of expected values is given by:

$$\frac{(\text{A x B})}{\text{C}}$$

First, we construct the table cross-tabulating the two variables.

In the new sheet labelled 'Chi sqrd':

- **Click** on A1.
- **Type** Actual values↵.
- **Click** on B2.
- **Type** Waiting time↵.
- **Click** on A3.
- **Type** Waiting area↵.
- **Click** on A4.
- **Type** Very satisfied↵.
- **Click** on A5.
- **Type** Quite satisfied↵.

🖰 **Click** on A6.

☛ **Type** No strong feelings ↵.

🖰 **Click** on A7.

☛ **Type** Quite dissatisfied↵.

🖰 **Click** on A7.

☛ **Type** Very dissatisfied↵.

🖰 **Click** on B3.

☛ **Type** Very satisfied↵.

🖰 **Click** on C3.

☛ **Type** Quite satisfied↵.

🖰 **Click** on D3.

☛ **Type** No strong feelings ↵.

🖰 **Click** on E3.

☛ **Type** Quite dissatisfied↵.

🖰 **Click** on F3.

☛ **Type** Very dissatisfied↵.

Hint: You may prefer to use copy and paste to copy the labels from the previous sheet.

We could use a complex compound statement based upon logical formulae acting on arrays to calculate the values required. However, we shall use a numerical shortcut.

To calculate the number of patients who were very satisfied with both the waiting time and the waiting area, we shall add together the responses to the second question and ten times the answer to the first question. This gives us a numerical value corresponding to each possible combination, shown in Table 7.8.

Table 7.8 Numerical values used to represent combinations.

Waiting time rating	*Waiting area rating*	*Numerical value*
Very satisfied (1)	Very satisfied (1)	11
	Quite satisfied (2)	12
	No strong feelings (3)	13
	Quite dissatisfied (4)	14
	Very dissatisfied (5)	15
Quite satisfied (2)	Very satisfied (1)	21
	Quite satisfied (2)	22
	No strong feelings (3)	23
	Quite dissatisfied (4)	24
	Very dissatisfied (5)	25
No strong feelings (3)	Very satisfied (1)	31
	Quite satisfied (2)	32
	No strong feelings (3)	33
	Quite dissatisfied (4)	34
	Very dissatisfied (5)	35
Quite dissatisfied (4)	Very satisfied (1)	41
	Quite satisfied (2)	42
	No strong feelings (3)	43
	Quite dissatisfied (4)	44
	Very dissatisfied (5)	45
Very dissatisfied (5)	Very satisfied (1)	51
	Quite satisfied (2)	52
	No strong feelings (3)	53
	Quite dissatisfied (4)	54
	Very dissatisfied (5)	55

Using this representation the formula required to produce the number of patients very satisfied with both waiting area and time becomes:

```
=SUM(IF('Main data'!$F$2:$F$734+('Main data'!$G$2:$G$734)*10=11,1,0))
```

In 'plain' English, this says:

> 'For each row between 2 and 734, calculate the sum of the value in column F and the ten times the value in column G. If this comes to eleven then add one to the running total, else add nothing.'

To implement this in practice:

- **Click** on B4.
- **Type** =SUM(IF('Main data'!$F$2:$F$734+('Main data'!$G$2:$G$734)*10=11,1,0)).

N.B. This should all be on the same line, it just doesn't fit!

- **Press** [Ctrl] and [⇧] and ↵ simultaneously to tell Excel that this is a compound statement.
- **Autofill** the formula across from B4 to F4.
- **Click** on C4.
- **Click** on the formula displayed at the top of the screen, immediately to the right of the =11.
- **Press** ←.
- **Type** 2.
- **Press** [Ctrl] and [⇧] and ↵ simultaneously to tell Excel that this is a compound statement.

In the same way, edit cells D4 to F4 to read as follows:

Cell D4:

=SUM(IF('Main data'!$F$2:$F$734+('Main data'!$G$2:$G$734)*10=13,1,0))

Cell E4:

=SUM(IF('Main data'!$F$2:$F$734+('Main data'!$G$2:$G$734)*10=14,1,0))

Cell F4:

=SUM(IF('Main data'!$F$2:$F$734+('Main data'!$G$2:$G$734)*10=15,1,0))

The correct values for this row of the table are given in Table 7.9 below.

Table 7.9 Calculated values for first row of table

Cell	*B4*	*C4*	*D4*	*E4*	*F4*
Value	1	19	27	32	86

To complete the table:

Paint B4 to F4.

Autofill the whole row down to B8 to F7.

Paint B5 to F5.

Select the Edit menu.

Select the Replace option.

Type =1 ⇥ =2.

Hint: The use of the = sign here allows us to distinguish between the 1 we wish to change and other 1s appearing in the fomula.

Click on [Replace All] to activate the replace option.

Paint B6 to F6.

Select the Edit menu.

Select the Replace option.

Type =1 ⇥ =3.

Click on [Replace All] to activate the replace option.

Paint B7 to F7.

Select the Edit menu.

Select the Replace option.

Type =1 ⇥ =4.

Click on [Replace All] to activate the replace option.

Paint B8 to F7.

Select the Edit menu.

Select the Replace option.

Type =1 ⇥ =5.

Click on [Replace All] to activate the replace option.

Next we need to calculate the row and column totals:

Click on G4.

Click on Σ.

Press ↵ to accept the formula.

Autofill down from G4 to G7.

Click on B9.

Click on Σ.

Press ↵ to accept the formula.

Autofill across from B9 to G9.

The completed table is illustrated below in Fig. 7.7:

	A	B	C	D	E	F	G
1	Actual values						
2		Waiting time					
3	Waiting Area	Very satis	Quite satis	No strong feel	Quite dissat	Very dissat	
4	Very satisfied	1	19	27	32	86	165
5	Quite satisfied	2	7	23	34	71	137
6	No strong feel	4	11	32	48	95	190
7	Quite dissatis	1	14	23	34	77	149
8	Very dissatis	0	11	13	27	41	92
9		8	62	118	175	370	733

Fig. 7.7 Completed table of actual values

Now we need to construct a table of values expected if there is no relationship between the factors. First we shall copy the labels:

Paint A3 to A8.

Click on .

Click on A13.

Click on .

Click on B2.

Click on .

Click on B12.

Click on .

- **Paint** B3 to F3.
- **Click** on .
- **Click** on B13.
- **Click** on .

Next, we shall enter the formulae in our table. Judicious use of dollar signs can save us a lot of work. The values are given by the product of the respective row and column totals divided by the overall total sample size.

- **Click** on B14.
- **Type** =$G4*B$9/$G$9↵.
- **Autofill** the formula across from B14 to F14.
- **Paint** B14 to F14
- **Autofill** the whole row down to B18 to F18.

The formulae required for the expected values table are illustrated in Fig. 7.8:

	B	C	D	E	F
12	Waiting time				
13	Very satisfied	Quite satisfied	No strong feelings	Quite dissatisfied	Very dissatisfied
14	=$G4*B$9/$G$9	=$G4*C$9/$G$9	=$G4*D$9/$G$9	=$G4*E$9/$G$9	=$G4*F$9/$G$9
15	=$G5*B$9/$G$9	=$G5*C$9/$G$9	=$G5*D$9/$G$9	=$G5*E$9/$G$9	=$G5*F$9/$G$9
16	=$G6*B$9/$G$9	=$G6*C$9/$G$9	=$G6*D$9/$G$9	=$G6*E$9/$G$9	=$G6*F$9/$G$9
17	=$G7*B$9/$G$9	=$G7*C$9/$G$9	=$G7*D$9/$G$9	=$G7*E$9/$G$9	=$G7*F$9/$G$9
18	=$G8*B$9/$G$9	=$G8*C$9/$G$9	=$G8*D$9/$G$9	=$G8*E$9/$G$9	=$G8*F$9/$G$9

Fig. 7.8 The formulae for the expected values table.

Now we'll format the cells to two decimal places:

- **Paint** B14 to F20.
- **Select** 'Format' from the menu bar.
- **Select** 'Cells'.
- **Select** the 'Number' category.
- **Select** 'Number'.
- **Select** '0.00'.

☛ **Press** ↵.

🖱 **Click** on A20.

☛ **Type** Chi-squared↵.

🖱 **Click** on B20.

☛ **Type** =CHITEST(B4:F8,B14:F18)↵.

The answer should be 0.58. The complete sheet is shown in Fig. 7.9.

	A	B	C	D	E	F	G
1	Actual values						
2		Waiting time					
3	Waiting Area	Very satis	Quite satis	No strong feel	Quite dissat	Very dissat	
4	Very satisfied	1	19	27	32	86	165
5	Quite satisfied	2	7	23	34	71	137
6	No strong feel	4	11	32	48	95	190
7	Quite dissatis	1	14	23	34	77	149
8	Very dissatis	0	11	13	27	41	92
9		8	62	118	175	370	733
10							
11	Expected val						
12		Waiting time					
13	Waiting Area	Very satis	Quite satis	No strong feel	Quite dissat	Very dissat	
14	Very satisfied	1.80	13.96	26.56	39.39	83.29	
15	Quite satisfied	1.50	11.59	22.05	32.71	69.15	
16	No strong feel	2.07	16.07	30.59	45.36	95.91	
17	Quite dissatis	1.63	12.60	23.99	35.57	75.21	
18	Very dissatis	1.00	7.78	14.81	21.96	46.44	
19							
20	Chi-squared	0.58					

Fig. 7.9 The final chi-squared sheet

This means that the probability of no relationship between these factors is relatively high. The dataset from this audit example contains much more information. We shall use it as the basis for a set of exercises which revise the lessons from this chapter and others.

7.3 COMPILING AN AUDIT REPORT

The next chapter illustrates how to put together a practice report based upon information from Excel. However, the final section provides tips on how to compile an audit report from this example.

7.4 EXERCISES

Each exercise should be tackled on a separate sheet within the audit workbook. A sample workbook including model solutions for each exercise is provided on the disk in the file 'solution.xls'.

1. Draw a pie chart showing the fraction of child patients amongst this study.

2. Sort the patient records by whether the patient is a child or not. Use the sorted version to calculate a new version of the frequency distributions, histograms and chi-squared tests for child patients only.

3. Calculate the waiting time between the request date and the appointment date. Using this sheet, calculate:

   a) the mean waiting time;
   b) the standard deviation of waiting times;
   c) the percentage of patients seen within 3, 6 and 12 months of the request date.

   Group the data into 3-month bands and plot a frequency histogram showing the distribution of waiting times for appointments.

4. Calculate the actual waiting time at the clinic from the difference between columns D and E. Group the data into 15-minute bands, i.e.

   up to 15 mins
   16-30 mins
   31-45 mins
   46-60 mins
   61-75 mins
   over 75 mins

Now carry out a chi-squared test to see whether there is a relationship between the actual waiting time and patients' satisfaction with the waiting time.

5. Repeat the chi-squared test in Q4 for child patients only.

8

Compiling reports

8.1 CHAPTER SUMMARY

Medical personnel are increasingly required to provide reports on performance. This requires linking data from many different sources. In this chapter, we shall continue the theme of medical audit and consider the problem of compiling an audit report drawn from a variety of sources.

In this chapter we shall cover the following issues:

- assembling a report from data in a range of sources;
- production of slides illustrating the main findings of the report.

The following features will be covered:

- importing data into Excel from other formats;
- linking applications and transporting data within the Windows environment;
- producing an audit report in Word for Windows to accommodate data and pictures from an Excel sheet;
- developing a presentation to support the written report.

8.2 THE PROBLEM

We have now seen the various ways in which Excel can be used to create budgets and plans together with charts and graphs which demonstrate the activities undertaken by health care professionals. Whilst these are useful, all too often the impact of such improvements through the use of Excel are not fully taken advantage of by users who are not acquainted with the ways in which such information can be fully and correctly incorporated into a word-processed document. The purpose of this chapter is to demonstrate how such spreadsheets and charts can be so incorporated into written documents using an application such as Word for Windows. In addition, we shall consider the problem of consolidating data from a number of sources.

The aim is not to teach Word for Windows or indeed any other package mentioned here but to demonstrate how better information can be provided through improved reports.

The medical audit under consideration has been carried out in the infertility clinic in Knapford General Hospital.

A medical audit has been conducted into the treatment of infertility at Knapford General Hospital. The study was conducted retrospectively on two parameters namely infertility investigations by all consultant firms within the Gynaecology Clinics and treatment within the Infertility Clinic.

To easily identify the infertility patients for the three consultant firms who do not have a specialized infertility clinic, the sample of patients was drawn from those who had undergone a test between the dates 1st January 1990 and 30th May 1991.

Concern had been expressed that the operational notes frequently contained insufficient information from the laparoscopy and dye procedure to be of use in the effective management of the patient's infertility. It was therefore decided to examine the case notes with a view to assessing the quality of information recorded in the operation notes and to examine what routine investigations were conducted.

A leading authority in the field has stated that in his opinion a laparoscopy and dye Test was the worst operation performed by the medical staff because of the wide range and varying skill of the operators, and inaccurate uninformative notes. It was his opinion that all laparoscopy and dye tests should be performed by the consultant or an operator of similar experience.

8.3 CONSOLIDATING INFORMATION

Our audit study combines data from a patient database together with information collected specifically for this audit, stored in an Excel 4.0 worksheet. We shall first combine them in an Excel 5.0 workbook.

The patient database is in Dbase III+ format and is called 'patients.dbf'. This contains clinical patient information. The Excel 4.0 worksheet is called 'infertil.xls' and contains information about the consulting firm and the status of the operator. We shall consolidate them into a workbook called 'audit3.xls'.

Click on .

At the Open dialog box,

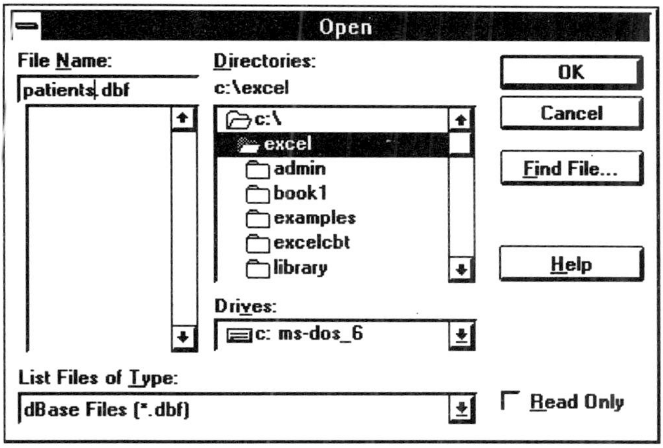

Fig. 8.1 The Open dialog box.

Type patients.dbf↵

The patient data is now on the screen.

Health Warning: Data may be imported in similar fashion from a wide range of formats such as Lotus 1-2-3, Quattro Pro and text-based formats such as tab-or comma-separated. You should always check the imported data for any quirks, as importation may be less than perfect.

The specific audit data may also be opened.

🖱 **Click** on .

☞ **Type** infertil.xls↵.

> **Hint**: This is no different from opening an Excel 5.0 workbook, so is identical to:
>
> 🖱 **Open** infertil.xls.

Now we can simply combine the two data sheets in one:

🖱 **Select** column B of 'infertil.xls'.

> **Hint**: To select the whole column, click on the header: 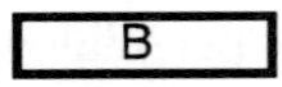
>

🖱 **Drag** across to select column C as well.

🖱 **Click** on .

🖱 **Select** 'patients.dbf' as the active worksheet.

🖱 **Select** column C.

🖱 **Select** 'Insert' from the menu bar.

🖱 **Select** 'Cut Cells'.

The extra information from infertil.xls is inserted into the patient data sheet. Note that all columns from C onwards move two columns to the right to accommodate the extra information.This is only possible because each data set identifies patients by the same unique identifying number.

Now we shall save our consolidated sheet:

🖱 **Select** 'File' from the menu bar.

🖱 **Select** 'Save As'.

☞ **Type** audit3.xls.

🖱 **Select** 'Excel workbook' as File type.

The completed dialog box is shown in Fig. 8.2.

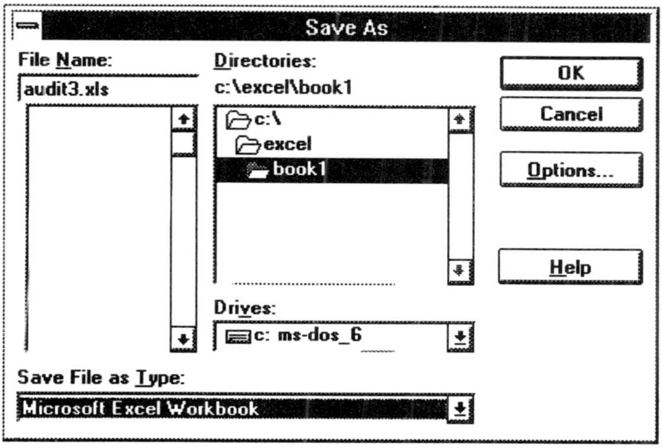

Fig. 8.2 The Save As dialog box.

Click on OK.

Select 'Window' from the menu bar.

Select 'infertil.xls'.

The modified sheet appears on the screen.

Select 'File' from the menu bar.

Select 'Close'.

Click on No, so that changes are **not** saved.

We are now left with a consolidated Excel sheet named 'patients', in a workbook called audit3.xls.

Minimize Excel.

> **Hint**: In future we shall use:
>
> **Minimize** Excel.
>
> To mean:
>
> **Click** on in the top right hand corner of the Excel application window.

Now we shall open our report in Word for Windows. The report, called audit3.doc, is stored in Word for Windows version 2.0 format.

This allows it to be read by both versions 2.0 and 6.0 of the package. From the Windows Program Manager:

🖰 **Click** on (version 2.0) or (version 6.0) to open Word for Windows.

Use to maximize the screen if necessary.

🖰 **Open** 'audit3.doc'.

> **Hint**: The Open operation works as in Excel:
>
> 🖰 **Click** on .
>
> 🖰 **Select** 'audit3.doc' (from the c:\winword directory).
>
> 🖰 **Click** on OK.

8.4 THE AUDIT REPORT

The picture shown in Fig. 8.3 could be created using the Draw facility within Excel. An alternative is to produce it in a Microsoft Draw which, in some respects, is easier to use as the cells of a spreadsheet in the background can be a distraction when using Excel.

This file has already been created in the word-processor. When the file is on the screen, locate the cursor right at the beginning and insert a page break:

Press [Ctrl] and [Home].

Press [Ctrl] and ↵.

On the first page we can now create the object to contain the picture.

🖰 **Select** 'Insert' from the menu bar.

🖰 **Select** 'Object'.

🖰 **Select** 'Microsoft Drawing'.

🖰 **Click** on OK.

Knapford General Hospital
KNAPFORD

KN1 4AW

MEDICAL AUDIT REPORT NO.3

1990-91

Fig. 8.3 The audit report cover.

We are now located in the Draw application, shown in Fig. 8.4. The main window is the area on which our picture will be drawn. On the left-hand side is a toolbar of tools associated with drawing. The pointer will change to other shapes according to the tool being used. At the bottom of the screen is a colour palette with line and fill options. The diamonds on the palette indicate that Line and/or Fill have been chosen for the colour associated with a drawing tool.

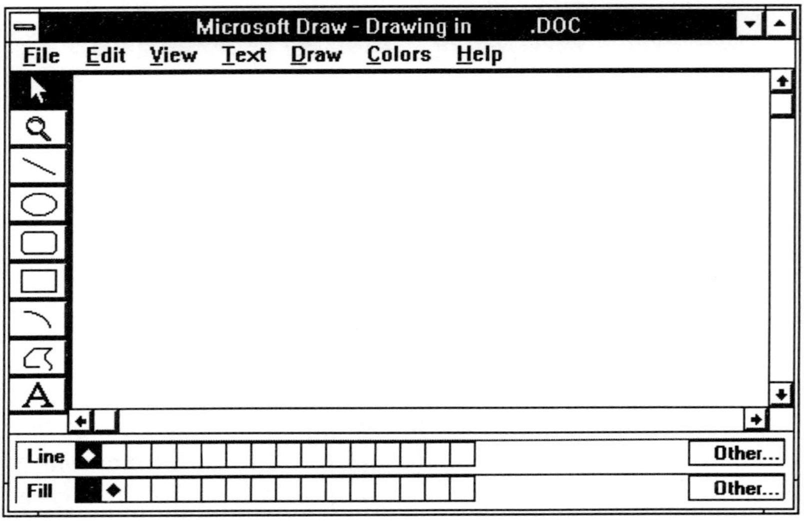

Fig. 8.4 The Microsoft Draw program.

The following section shows how the picture above has been created. Follow the instructions to replicate this picture or create your own.

- **Click** on the black square for Line and Fill on the Colour Palette.
- **Click** on 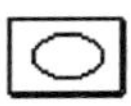, the circle on the toolbar.
- **Move** the cross-hairs icon to centre screen.
- **Drag** the Mouse until a circle appears and release the left mouse button.

A black circle should appear. Now we shall use the following procedure to create a semi-circle.

- **Click** on 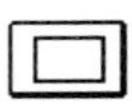, the rectangle .
- **Click** on the white square for Line and Fill on the colour palette.

Move the cross-hair to half way down the left side of the circle.

Drag across and down to blot out the lower half of the circle so that only the black upper half remains. Now for the pillars.

Click on 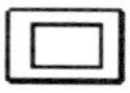, the rectangle.

Click on the black square for Line and Fill on the Palette.

Move and **drag** to create a small pillar below the Semi-Circle.

This can now be copied using the Edit and Copy function to create the other pillars.

Click on the pillar.

Select 'Edit' from the menu bar.

Select 'Copy'.

Select 'Edit' from the menu bar.

Select 'Paste'.

A duplicated pillar will now appear from where it can be moved by Dragging to an appropriate location. Repeat the exercise to produce four pillars in total. Create the baubles on top of the dome in the same way as the circle was first created. Oval shapes will be created simply by appropriate movements of the mouse. To create the church spire:

Click on 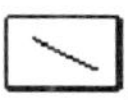, the diagonal line in the toolbar.

Move and drag for each component part of the line to be created. Finally we can add text. This could be left out at this stage with the text being added later in the Word for Windows document, but if you wish to use the object created for letterheads and other purposes, it might be worthwhile adding the text here with the text drawing tool.

Click 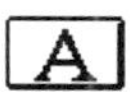 in the toolbar to create text.

We shall need to determine the font and size of text:

Select 'Text' from the menu bar.

Select 'Font'.

Select 'Times New Roman'.

Select 'Text' from the menu bar.

🖱 **Select** 'Size'.

🖱 **Select** '14'.

Position the 'bar' icon at an appropriate point above the drawing and type in the name of the hospital. If it is not quite in the right place, it can be moved later. For the title 'Medical Audit Report, No. 3, 1990-1', choose a larger typeface.

🖱 **Select** 'Text' from the menu bar.

🖱 **Select** 'Size'.

🖱 **Select** '18'.

🖱 **Position** the bar icon.

☛ **Type** 'Medical Audit Report No.3' ↵

🖱 **Position** the bar icon.

☛ **Type** '1990-91'.

If you make a mistake at any point the Edit and Cut facility can be used once an object has been selected. If you need to move an object to a different position, simply hold down the left mouse button and drag. The image required has now been created. It can be saved in the following manner:

🖱 **Select** 'File' from the menu bar.

🖱 **Select** 'Update'.

🖱 **Select** 'File' from the menu bar.

🖱 **Select** 'Exit and Return to Document'.

> **Hint:** This is the first example of embedding an object. In this case the object is a Microsoft Draw graphic. We shall return to this topic later.

The object will now appear in the document and can be saved as a component of the document. Although it is attached to this particular document, it can always be copied and pasted to other documents.

Next we shall move to the text of the report itself.

8.5 INCORPORATING DATA AND CHARTS FROM EXCEL IN THE AUDIT REPORT

The first page of text is an introduction which describes the audit study. On the next page we find the data describing the overall number of procedures:

INFERTILITY INVESTIGATIONS

DATA REPORT

Total number of laparoscopy and dye test procedures undertaken in 1989 = 133

Table 1: Procedures undertaken by consultant firm

Brown,11
Davis,97
Evans,13
Smith,12

The table is currently displayed as comma-delimited. This is a quick way of putting in data which we want to display as a table. This may easily be displayed as a table:

- **Paint** the four lines of text.
- **Select** 'Table' from the menu bar.
- **Select** 'Convert Text to Table'.
- In Word 6.0, **Click** on [OK].

and Word will turn the data into a table:

Brown	11
Davis	97
Evans	13
Smith	12

We must then decide upon the format for the table. With the table still highlighted:

- **Click** on 'Format'.
- **Click** on 'Border'.
- **Click** on 'Grid'.
- **Click** on OK.

The table now looks like:

Brown	11
Davis	97
Evans	13
Smith	12

Now we can reduce the column widths by dragging the boundaries much as we used to in Excel. The final result should look like

Brown	11
Davis	97
Evans	13
Smith	12

Table 2 may be reconstructed in much the same way. Try it as an exercise. Change:

Table 2: Sample for this audit

*Davis,20
Brown,16
Evans,19
Smith,16
Waiting list initiative,11
Registrar list ,2

into:

Table 2: Sample for this audit

*Davis	20
Brown	16
Evans	19
Smith	16
Waiting list initiative	11
Registrar list	2

We shall construct the next table from the data stored in our Excel sheet.

8.5.1 Copying and pasting

With Windows applications it is possible to copy and paste not only within an application but between applications. This is performed by using what is known as the 'clipboard'. The clipboard itself is a Windows application which can be opened from the Program Manager Accessories when you see this icon:

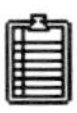

When a group of cells in a worksheet or part of a chart or picture are cut or copied, they are automatically placed in the clipboard which retains them even when the application itself is closed down.

Hint: If a large amount of data is placed in the clipboard, Windows will ask you whether you wish to keep the data in the clipboard after the application has been shut down.

Click on [Yes] if you don't wish to lose the data.

It is then simply a question of pasting those items into a new document when Word for Windows is opened. The procedure is as follows:

Minimize Word.

If Excel is currently mimimized:

Double-click on the Excel icon 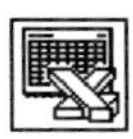.

Excel will now be back on the screen. First, we shall calculate the values needed in the table, then we shall import them. Enter the formulae shown in Fig. 8.5 to calculate the required values:

- **Click** on A100.
- **Type** Primary↵.
- **Type** Secondary↵.
- **Type** Not infertility↵.
- **Click** on B102.
- **Type** =COUNTA(A2:A93)-COUNTA(B2:B93).
- **Click** on B101.
- **Type** =SUM(B2:B93)-COUNTA(B2:B93).
- **Click** on B100.
- **Type** =COUNTA(B2:B93)-B101.

Hint: It is easier if you enter the formulae in reverse order: row 102 first, then 101, then 100.

	A	B
100	Primary	=COUNTA(B2:B93)-B101
101	Secondary	=SUM(B2:B93)-COUNTA(B2:B93)
102	Not infertility	=COUNTA(A2:A93)-COUNTA(B2:B93)

Fig. 8.5 Formulae to be entered.

Next we shall paste the data from Excel into Word:

- **Paint** A100 to B102.
- **Click** on .
- **Minimize** Excel.
- **Maximize** Word.
- **Click** on the document below the header for Table 3.
- **Click** on .

Now the table appears in the Word document.
Next, resize and format it as for Tables 1 and 2. The final results should look like:

Table 3 Infertility classification

Primary	50
Secondary	34
Not infertility	8

In the next section we need to record the range of values for the duration of infertility and the mean value:

Duration of infertility

The stated duration of the infertility to the first appointment with the Consultant where the complaint was 'infertility' ranged from between__and___months with a mean of___months. The duration was not stated in 9 case records.

Once again, we calculate the values in the sheet:

- **Minimize** Word.
- **Maximize** Excel.
- **Click** on C94.
- **Type** =MIN(C2:C93)↵.
- **Type** =MAX(C2:C93)↵
- **Type** =AVERAGE (C2:C93)↵

Now we can copy these values into our text:

- **Click** on C94.
- **Click** on .
- **Minimize** Excel.
- **Maximize** Word.
- **Click** on the document after the word 'between'.
- **Click** on .

Repeat for the maximum value and average value pasting them in at the appropriate point. You may like to format them to match the rest of the document. To do this:

- **Paint** the number to be changed.
- **Click** on the point size box.
- **Type** 12↵.

The next paragraph requires the number of operations carried out by Consultant firms and the breakdown by operator:

of the operations were performed by Consultant firms; the breakdown of the status of the operator is:

Table 4: Operator status

To calculate the total number of operations carried out by the consultant firms, enter the following formula into D94:

- **Click** on D94.
- **Type** =COUNT(D2:D93)↵.

The resulting value could now be copied and pasted into the document. However, let us suppose we wish instead to link the value in the document to the value in the spreadsheet. This has the advantage that if the data in the sheet changes, so the figure in the report will be updated.

8.5.2 Object linking

The process of copying and pasting described above is the easiest to follow but has the disadvantage that data cannot be changed except manually or by re-importing the data. If data is being produced at the last minute before the report is complete, with substantial portions of the document already finished, it can be quite tedious to change items manually or to re-import. There is also a danger that the data imported may be incorrect. A better method is to use the Object Linking facility. An object may be anything from a single figure to a complete Excel workbook.

To object link a number of procedures:

- **Click** on D94.
- **Click** on .
- **Minimize** Excel.
- **Maximize** Word.
- **Click** on the document at the start of the paragraph.
- **Click** on the 'Edit' in the menu bar.
- **Click** on 'Paste Special'.
- **Click** on [Paste Link].

Ensure that the format is selected as 'Rich Text Format'.

- **Click** on [OK].

The result appears the same as an ordinary paste but as the sheet is updated, so the figure updates too. Links may be used between Excel sheets, too.

To fill out Table 5 we can create a linked spreadsheet within our audit3.xls workbook, then link the results to Table 5 in Word.

- **Minimize** Word.
- **Maximize** Excel.
- **Paint** the range C1 to D93.
- **Click** on .
- **Select** 'Insert' from the menu bar.
- **Select** 'Worksheet'.
- **Select** 'Edit' from the menu bar.
- **Select** 'Paste Special'.
- **Click** on [Paste Link].

The cells A1 to B93 are now linked to cells C1 to D93.

- **Click** on C2.
- **Type** =IF($A2=1,IF($B2="C",1,0),0).
- **Autofill** the formula down as far as C93.

- **Click** on C94.
- **Click** on [Σ].
- **Press** ↵.

This is the number of patients who had their operations performed by the consulting firm headed by Dr Brown and carried out by the consultant himself.

- **Click** on D2.
- **Type** =IF($A2=1,IF($B2="R",1,0),0).
- **Autofill** the formula down as far as D93.
- **Click** on D94.
- **Click** on [Σ].
- **Press** ↵.

This is the number of patients who had their operations performed by the consulting firm headed by Dr Brown and a registrar. Repeat this process using the following formulae:

Table 8.1 Formulae for cells E2 to N2

Cell	*Formula*
E2	=IF($A2=1,IF($B2="S",1,0),0)
F2	=IF($A2=2,IF($B2="C",1,0),0)
G2	=IF($A2=2,IF($B2="R",1,0),0)
H2	=IF($A2=2,IF($B2="S",1,0),0)
I2	=IF($A2=3,IF($B2="C",1,0),0)
J2	=IF($A2=3,IF($B2="R",1,0),0)
K2	=IF($A2=3,IF($B2="S",1,0),0)
L2	=IF($A2=4,IF($B2="C",1,0),0)
M2	=IF($A2=4,IF($B2="R",1,0),0)
N2	=IF($A2=4,IF($B2="S",1,0),0)

- **Click** on C94.
- **Click** on .
- **Minimize** Excel.
- **Maximize** Word.
- **Click** on the first blank cell of Table 5.
- **Click** on the 'Edit' in the menu bar.
- **Click** on 'Paste Special'.
- **Click** on [Paste Link].

Ensure that the format is selected as 'Rich Text Format'.

- **Click** on [OK].

Complete the table by using paste link:

Firm	Consultants	Reg	SHO
Brown	Link to C94	Link to D94	Link to E94
Davis	Link to F94	Link to G94	Link to H94
Evans	Link to I94	Link to J94	Link to K94
Smith	Link to L94	Link to M94	Link to N94

There is more data in the workbook and more of the report to fill in, but this is left for you to investigate.

8.6 NOTES ON PRODUCING OHPS

Often it is desirable to back up a written report with a verbal presentation. To support such a presentation, a set of overhead projection slides can be produced, hereafter referred to as OHP slides. This may be done using a specialist presentation package such as Powerpoint, Freelance or Harvard Graphics. It is, however, possible to produce slides using just a word processor if no presentation package is available or familiar to the user.

In this section we shall show how OHP slides may be created. Rather than discuss a specific package we shall consider a general approach to the problem.

The overall approach is shown in Fig. 8.6. Whichever package is used, the approach is the same. First prepare your template in the presentation package of your choice.

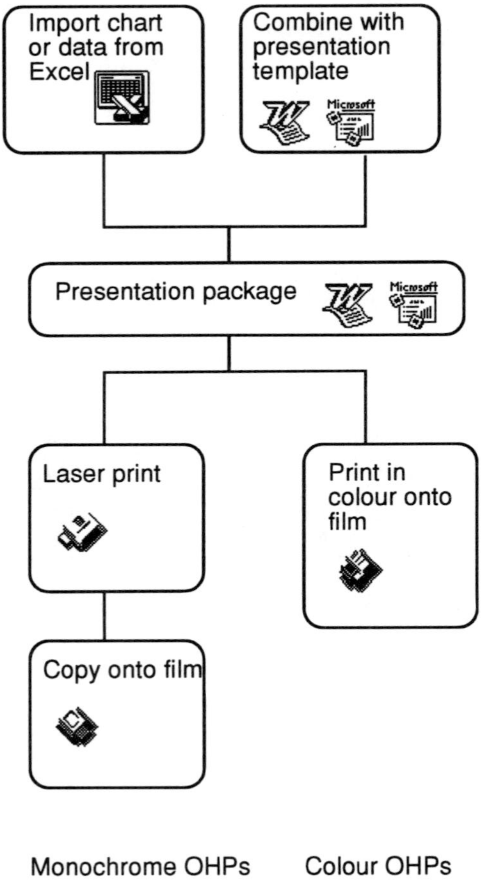

Fig. 8.6 An approach to preparing OHPs.

The sample disk contains two template files, house.dot and house.ppt, which are applicable to Word and Powerpoint respectively. House.dot is shown in Fig. 8.7 and a sample slide illustrated in Fig. 8.8.

Medical Audit, No.3

Infertility Clinic, Knapford General Hospital

Presented by: **Slide No:**

Fig. 8.7 The House.dot house style template.

The approach recommended will be illustrated with Word for Windows, but a similar approach may be applied with any of the specialist presentation packages:

- **Select** ‘File’ from the menu bar.
- **Select** ‘New’.
- **Select** ‘house’ from the list of templates.

Now return to Excel, to sheet1 within the audit3.xls workbook.

- **Click** on B95.
- **Type** =SUM(IF(B2:B93=“C”,1,0)).
- **Press** [Ctrl] and [⇧] and ↵.
- **Click** on B96.
- **Type** =SUM(IF(B2:B93=“R”,1,0)).
- **Press** [Ctrl] and [⇧] and ↵.
- **Click** on B97.
- **Type** =SUM(IF(B2:B93=“S”,1,0)).
- **Press** [Ctrl] and [⇧] and ↵.
- **Paint** B95 to B97.

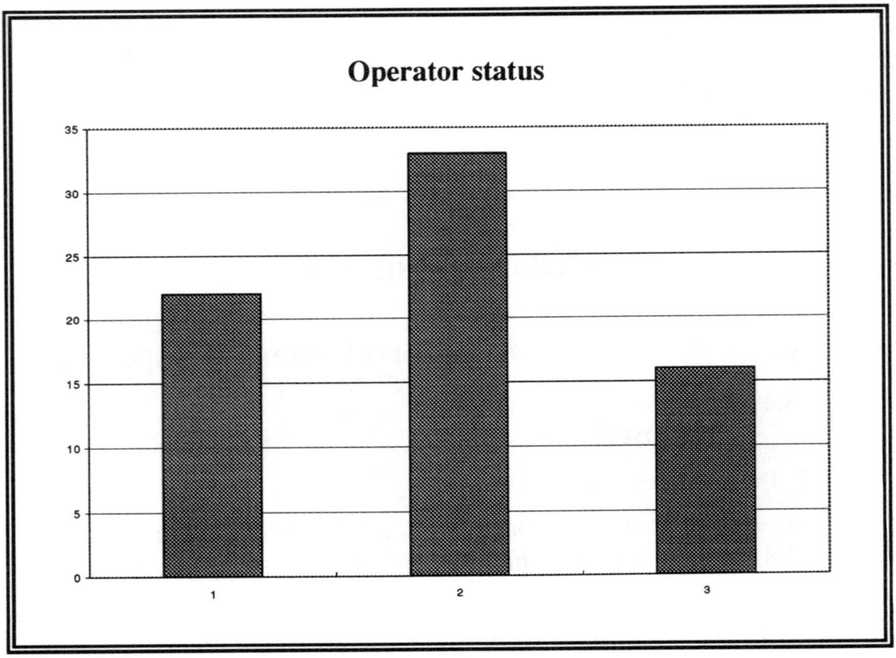

Medical Audit, No.3

Infertility Clinic, Knapford General Hospital

Presented by: Dr Brown **Slide No: 3**

Fig. 8.8 A sample OHP slide.

- ☛ **Press** [F11] to construct a column chart on a new sheet.
- 🖱 Tailor the appearance of the chart using the ChartWizard.
- 🖱 **Select** the whole chart.
- 🖱 **Click** on .
- 🖱 **Minimize** Excel.
- 🖱 **Maximize** Word.

Return to Word:

- 🖱 **Click** on .
- 🖱 **Select** the chart within the Word document.
- 🖱 **Select** 'Format' from the menu bar.
- 🖱 **Select** 'Border'.
- 🖱 **Select** 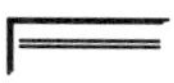.
- 🖱 **Click** on 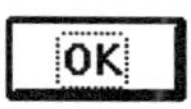.
- ☛ Complete the presenter and slide number details.

This general approach may be used whatever the presentation package. If the desired result is monochrome, then the easiest way to achieve high quality results is to print out the slides on a laser printer and then photocopy the results onto OHP film. If a colour printer is available, then it may better to print the results straight onto OHP film in colour.

8.7 OBJECT EMBEDDING

As the above has demonstrated, it can be quite tedious moving back and forth between applications even when dynamic data exchange is employed. Occasionally a simple change is needed to data or the addition of some minor element to a chart. Embedding an object within a document allows the possibility of editing the elements within the object while remaining in the document. For example, we may wish to alter the legend within the chart just produced.

When we cut and paste a chart from Excel into a Word document, it is actually embedded as a picture object. If you now click on the chart in the Word document, then you are automatically in the drawing program to allow you to tailor the appearance of the chart. Note that as the chart is embedded as a picture object rather than an Excel 5.0 chart, you cannot edit the underlying data in this way.

Another example of an embedded object is the front cover, which is a Microsoft Drawing Object embedded in its own format. Thus we can double-click on it and have full access to all aspects of the picture.

If you want to embed the Excel workbook itself to allow full access to the information, then you should proceed as follows:

> **Hint**: The following procedure works with Word 6.0. Word 2.0 has a similar but not identical procedure.

- **Select** 'Insert' from the menu bar.
- **Select** 'Object'.
- **Select** [Create from File].

From the resulting dialog box, shown in Fig. 8.9:

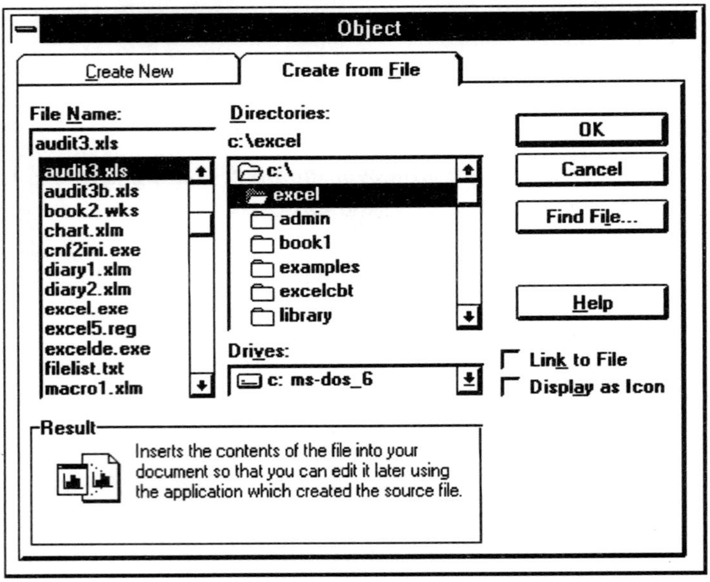

Fig. 8.9 The Insert Object dialog box.

- **Select** 'audit3.xls'.

The worksheet now appears as an icon: 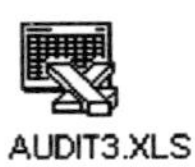

Double-click on the icon to run the Excel application from within the document.

> **Health Warning:** Linking and embedding is very attractive, but is very resource intensive. Do not use it unless there is a good reason for doing so.

9

Disasters! And how to avoid them

9.1 CHAPTER SUMMARY

You may have just lost all your data through a mishap with your computer. At this point, it is unfortunately too late to prevent the mishap. In this chapter we shall allow you to travel back prior to the disaster to see what you should have done to prevent it. If you have survived this far and are tempted to omit this chapter, remember you have been warned!

The topics included in this chapter include:

- prevention of disasters resulting in loss of data;
- viruses and their prevention;
- disk tracking to allow recovery of deleted files;
- legal requirements.

Features covered in Excel and the Windows environment include:

- security features within Excel;
- use of file attributes to protect files;
- good housekeeping practices including backups.

9.2 DOCUMENT AND CELL PROTECTION

Once a document has been completed it is easy to overwrite it in some way by accident. It can however, be protected either at the level of the document as a whole or at the level of the individual cells.

9.2.1 Document protection

To protect the whole document:

- **Select** 'Tools' from the menu bar.
- **Select** 'Protection'.
- **Select** 'Protect Sheet'.

The sheet may be protected without using a password. If you require the additional protection of a password, enter it at this stage.

- **Type** a password (and remember it!).
- **Click** on [OK].

The document as a whole cannot now be changed unless the option to unprotect the document is used. This is a good way to protect sensitive data, e.g. patient records, but if you forget your password, then it will be protected even from you!

9.2.2 Cell protection

In many instances, the whole sheet needs to be protected except for certain portions of it. You may, for example, want to protect the logic of a sheet which contains all your budget calculations, but vary the data. This would enable you to carry out scenario analysis to calculate 'what happens if' or use the sheet year after year with only a change in annual data.

Cells are automatically 'locked' in order to ensure that they cannot be changed when the sheet as a whole is protected. In order to unlock the cells containing data, the following procedure should be used:

- **Paint** a row containing data.
- **Select** 'Format'.

Select 'Cells'.

Click on ☒ to unlock the cells.

Click on OK.

9.2.3 Password protection

Besides the methods used above, it is possible to use password protection at two levels within Excel. The first level involves general protection of the worksheet:

Select 'File' from the menu bar.

Select 'Save As'.

Select 'Options'.

Type a protection password.

Re-type the password to confirm.

Click on OK.

Save the file in the usual way. When the file is next retrieved, the correct password will have to be provided in order to use the worksheet.

9.2.4 Write protection

The method above protects in a general way. It is also possible to provide write password protection. This will allow the data to be viewed but not permanently changed.

Select 'File' from the menu bar.

Select 'Save As'.

Select 'Options'.

Type in a write reservation password.

Click on OK.

Re-type the write reservation password

Click on OK.

Save the file in the usual way.

When the file is subsequently retrieved, a password will be required to use it in 'write reservation' mode. If the user does not know the password it can still be used in 'read-only' mode. It will be possible to alter the sheet – both figures and formulae. However, if one attempts to save the file, a message indicating the file is 'read-only' will appear.

It is possible to use password protection and write reservation protection in combination.

9.2.5 Changing file attributes in Excel and File Manager

It is possible to make worksheets 'read-only' from within Excel. This can be achieved when a file is ready to be saved. A worksheet which is 'read-only' cannot be edited or amended and it cannot be deleted.

Select 'File' from the main menu of Excel.

Select 'Save as'.

Select 'Options'.

Click on ☒ Read Only Recommended.

Click on [OK].

Name the file as appropriate.

Click on [OK] to save the file.

There are a number of facilities which can be used within the Windows environment which afford a certain amount of protection to files which have been created. If you have not protected the worksheet within Excel it is possible to protect it from the File Manager.
In order to use them use the following procedure:

Select File Manager from the Windows Applications screen.

Select a file to protect.

Hint: Use the Search option if you have a number of files and one you want is not immediately to hand.

Select 'Properties'.

Read-only files.

Files can be made 'read-only': a user may read the file but is not allowed to edit or amend the file. This also implies that the file cannot be deleted.

🖰 **Click** on ☒ Read Only.

🖰 **Click** on OK.

Health Warning: Whichever way you protect the sheet, unprotect it when required by using the same facility.

9.2.6 Hidden files

Files can also be hidden, i.e. they will not appear on the general listing of files and therefore will be hidden from the view of the user. The person making the file hidden will, however, be in a position to cause the files to be displayed when required. From the same 'Properties' menu:

🖰 **Click** on ☒ Hidden.

9.3 GOOD HOUSEKEEPING

9.3.1 Saving twice

One of the major losses of data is through accidental deletion or corruption of files. It is not always possible to avoid such a situation but the aim must be to recover from it as quickly as possible. In the examples we have used, it is possible to save the worksheets to one or more floppy disks separately as well as to the hard disk. It is best to get into a routine of saving work to the floppy disk immediately after saving to the hard disk or, at least, at the end of a work session.

9.3.2 Using directories

Often worksheets are not lost at all even though the user claims this to be the case. Disorganization of data on the disk can result in the apparent loss of data and files. Worksheets can be organized on the disk using appropriate directories to store data according to its usage, e.g. all Excel workbooks held together and all worksheets in workbooks associated with specific projects or tasks.

The Create Directory option within Windows File Manager can be used to create appropriate directories for your work. The systems available within Windows can work for you to create an ordered environment.

Disks may be both physically and logically labelled in order to help the process of ensuring no 'loss' of data. The label should of course be the same. Disks may labelled from the File Manager. The File Manager facilities were covered in Chapter One.

9.3.4 Backing Up

Where large amounts of data are involved – usually well beyond the storage of worksheets, then other means of backing up work created must be considered. There are two possibilities. Floppy disks may be used in conjunction with the Backup command within DOS to store reasonable amounts of data, but the operation can become tedious if large amounts of data are involved, for example a backup which involved more than two or three floppy disks. The Restore command in DOS can be used subsequently to re-load the lost data if necessary.

The process of data storage can be facilitated by the use of data compression packages, creating 'Zip' files, which will reduce the amount of data down to a level only about 10% to 15% of the original volume. However, for really large amounts of data, such as may be kept on the patient record system in the surgery, tape backup is recommended and should be carried out on a regular basis. Evidence from general practices suggest that this is not being done regularly and, in some cases, the consequences of not doing so could be potentially disastrous for any practice. Hospital clinics are just the same.

If you have DOS version 6.0 or above, then there is a useful backup facility provided under Windows. It should be accessible either from the Program Manager or from the Tools menu in the File Manager.

Backing up is not glamorous, but can save your data (Fig. 9.1).

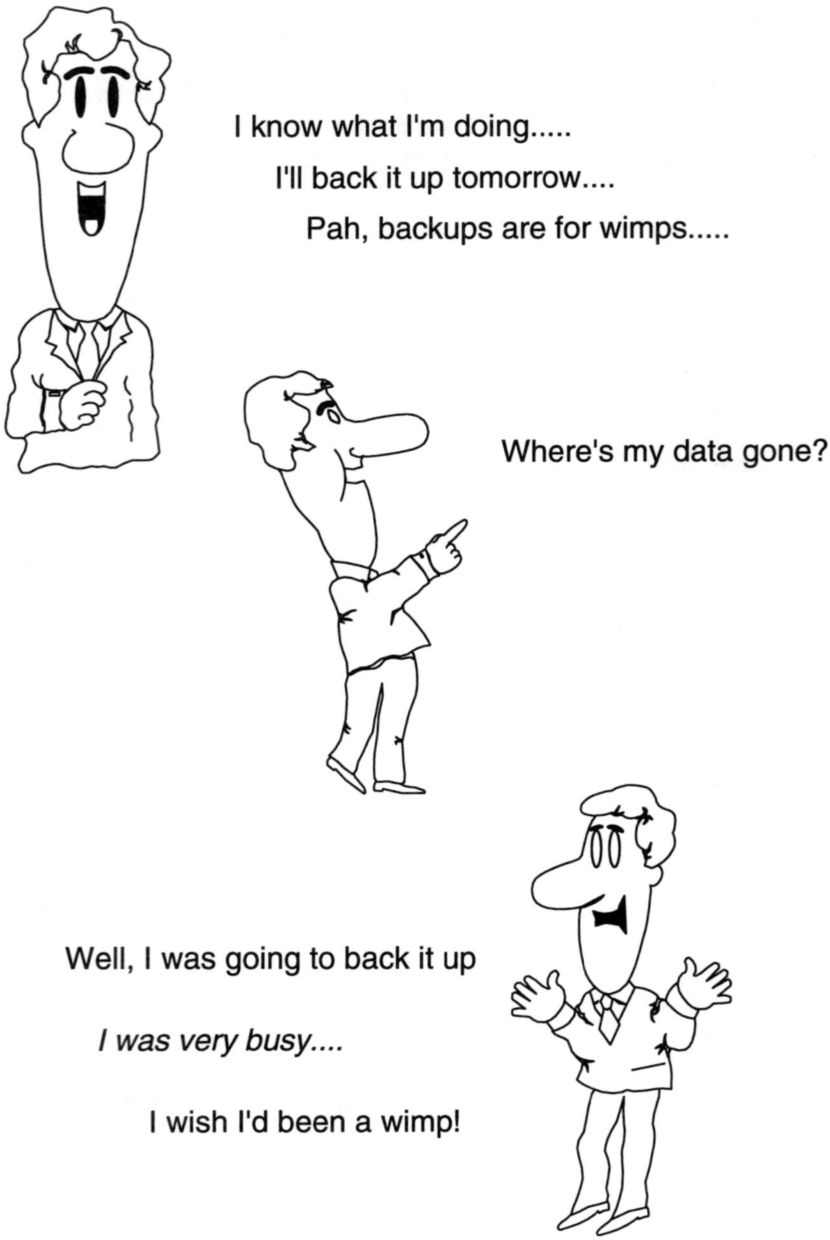
I know what I'm doing.....
I'll back it up tomorrow....
Pah, backups are for wimps.....
Where's my data gone?
Well, I was going to back it up
I was very busy....
I wish I'd been a wimp!

Fig. 9.1 A cautionary tale...

9.4. VIRUSES

Computer viruses are simply computer programs which result in unexpected and unwanted effects in the computer system. At their most harmless, they produce unwanted tricks; at their most harmful, they can destroy all the data, i.e. all your patients records on the hard disk of your system.

Computer viruses are contracted, i.e. spread to your computer system in one of two ways, either through floppy disks which have the viral program stored on them or by being downloaded from a computer elsewhere though a computer network. The former is far more likely than the latter. The usual way the originator of a virus causes the spread is through attaching the virus software code to another programme. When the program is copied from the floppy disk, so is the virus.

It is not surprising that games software is the most likely source of virus infections. Like some natural viruses, there are ways of avoiding them. Just as most transmission of HIV or hepatitis occurs through known and avoidable practices such as unsafe sex or the sharing needles amongst drug addicts, so safe practice can protect you from computer viruses. If you do not share disks (the most common way of viral spread), you cannot contract them! Of course, good practices must be followed by all users of the computer system.

Doctors should, therefore, be in an excellent position to understand this. Software producers and floppy disk manufacturers ensure that their software and disks are free from viruses at the point of manufacture. Legally purchased software will therefore have a minimal risk as will blank disks.

Anti-viral software can be purchased from a number of sources. It comes in two forms. The first type will detect all known viruses and report which viruses are present either in memory or on the hard disk. There are, of course, new viruses being developed by malicious programmers. The second type of software will eradicate the virus from the system. There are fewer examples of this type so although the virus detector may be able to detect the virus, it may not be able to remove it. It is useful to have anti-virus software on the system. If data does have to be shared between systems where the source may not always be known, a floppy can be scanned by the anti-viral software to report the presence or absence of a virus. If the disk is virus-free, the files can then be copied on to the hard disk.

DOS 6.0 and subsequent versions provides its own virus protection utility. Many reviews suggest that the level of protection provided is less than ideal. However, it is clearly better than nothing. Once again, if it is present on your machine, there will be a tools menu within the File Manager.

9.5. LEGAL REQUIREMENTS

9.5.1 Data Protection Act 1984

Since 1984, data concerning individuals which is kept electronically is subject to the Data Protection Act. The following provides an outline of the issues concerned with data protection and how it operates with respect to health care. Further information can be obtained from the Data Protection Registrar.

9.5.2 Purpose

The purpose of the Act is to protect the rights of individuals in respect of the information recorded about them on computer. Any individual, known as the Data Subject, has the right to find out about any data kept about him/her and in certain cases, challenge that data, for example in respect of accuracy, and claim compensation. There is often confusion about what data the Act actually covers. Any automatically processed information relating to any living identifiable individual comes within the sphere of the Act. Since many types of equipment automatically process information, the coverage is wider than computers alone. The Act covers statements of fact about that individual, e.g. an address and expressions of opinion e.g. than an individual is honest and trustworthy, but does not cover intentions e.g. X will be promoted next month. Exemptions include personal data used for paying wages and pensions; keeping accounts; records of purchases and sales; personal data used for distribution e.g. names and addresses. However, in the latter case, there is no exemption if an objection is made. Publicly published data sources, such as the electoral register, are also exempt.

All organizations or individuals holding personal data must register as Data Users with the Data Protection Registrar. The entry in the register must indicate the personal data held; the purpose for which it is held; the sources of the data; the people to whom it will be disclosed; and whether it will be transferred abroad.

9.5.3 Principles

There are a number of principles upon which the keeping of personal data is allowed:

- Fair and lawful processing

The first is that the processing of any personal data should be done fairly and lawfully.

- Lawful purpose.

The data kept on an individual should not be for any illegal purpose - for example, the perpetration of a fraud on that individual.

- Adequate.
- Relevant and not excessive.

The information should only be relevant to the purpose for which it is kept and cannot be kept for any incidental purpose. If data is kept for medical purposes, it cannot be used for any other purpose. No data should be kept which is unnecessary for that purpose. For example, bank account details are irrelevant and are excessive for medical purposes.

- Accurate and up-to-date.

For any organization, this can be a major problem but accuracy is important under the Act. Information indicating that a patient has a medical problem which they do not in fact have can obviously be detrimental to that individual. It may also be that one diagnosis has been superseded by a second. If the first diagnosis is the only one on record, then that personal information is obviously not up-to-date.

- Minimum period held.

Data should only be kept whilst it is needed. It should therefore be kept for as short a time as necessary. Obviously, in the case of medical records, this will involve a patient's lifetime. However, in the case of a patient who has moved away and registered with another practice, data should be kept no longer than is necessary to effect a smooth transfer of records.

- Security.

The data must be kept secure from access by any unauthorised individual who is not the data user. This implies that physical security in the practice should be good, that no individual in the practice should have access to it unless as part of their work, that all systems should be password protected and that there should be secure networks if data is downloaded from a remote source. Data security is likely to be a major problem in the future with so much information being held by hospitals and practices. Advice should be sought from hospital computer services or from Family Health Service Authorities.

Any Data Subject about whom data is kept has the right of access to any data and can demand correction or deletion in the case of inaccuracy and may merit compensation.

9.5.4 Summary of data protection requirements

If you keep patient records on computer, then you are almost certainly required to register under the Data Protection Act. Although all parts of the NHS are likely to be registered, a regional survey found almost 90% of general practice registrations to be inadequate within the geographical area under consideration. As your information changes, so this should be reflected in your data protection registration. If in doubt, contact the Data Protection Registrar.

Appendix

MENU BAR COMMANDS

Table A.1 shows the correspondence between commands selected from the menu bar in Excel version 5.0 and commands in Excel version 4.0. This is not an exhaustive list but contains all those used in this book.

TOOLBAR BUTTONS

Tables A.2 and A.3 show the toolbar buttons associated with the standard and formatting toolbars respectively. The tables only show the buttons referred to in this text, and then only when they have been added since version 4.0. The tables show where there is an equivalent menu command in version 4.0 or where there is no equivalent at all.

Many more toolbar buttons are available by using the customizing facilities in version 5:

Select 'View' from the menu bar.

Select 'Toolbars'.

Click on 'Customize'.

Select a category from the 'Categories' list.

Drag the chosen icon to the toolbar of your choice.

See Chapter 6 for an example.

Most of the buttons on the version 5.0 formatting toolbar have equivalent functions under the Toolbars option on the Options menu in version 4.0.

Table A.1 **Menu bar commands**

Version 5.0	*Version 4.0*
File Menu	***File Menu***
Save	Save Workbook
	Options Menu
Sheet Tab, Page Setup	Set Print Area
Sheet Tab, Page Setup	Set Print Titles
Edit Menu	***Edit Menu***
Paste Special	Paste Link
Fill, Right	Fill Right
Fill, Down	Fill Down
	Formula Menu
Go To	Go To
Find	Find
Replace	Replace
	Data Menu
Delete Row	Delete
	Format Menu
Fill, Justify	Justify
	Data Menu
Fill, Series	Series
View Menu	***Options Menu***
Toolbars	Toolbars
Color Tab, Options	Color Palette
Protection, Protect Workbook and Unprotect Workbook	Protect Document
Protection, Protect Sheet and Unprotect Sheet	Protect Document
Options, Calculation Tab,	Calculation
Spelling	Spelling
Data Analysis	Analysis Tools
Insert Menu	***Edit Menu***
Cells	Insert
Rows	Insert
Columns	Insert
Object	Insert Object

Table A.1 Menu bar commands (cont'd)

	Formula Menu
Name,Paste	Paste Name
Function	Paste Function
Name,Define	Define Name
Name,Create	Create Names
Name,Apply	Apply Names
Note	Note
Format Menu	***Format Menu***
Number Tab, Cells	Number
Alignment Tab, Cells	Alignment
Font Tab, Cells	Font
Border Tab, Cells	Border
Patterns Tab, Cells	Patterns
Protection Tab, Cells	Cell Protection
Row	Row Height
Column	Column Width
Tools Menu	***Formula Menu***
Goal Seek	Goal Seek
Scenarios	Scenario Manager
Solver	Solver
	Options Menu
View Tab, Options	Display
	Macro Menu
Macro	Run
Record Macro, Record New Macro	Record
Data Menu	***Data Menu***
Filter	Find
PivotTable	Crosstab
View Menu	***Window Menu***
View Manager	View
Zoom	Zoom

Table A.2 Standard toolbar

Version 5.0	*Version 4.0*
	Print, Preview
	No equivalent
	Edit, Redo
	Data, Sort, Ascending
	Options, Toolbars
	Options, Spelling
	Edit, Undo
	Formula
	Data, Sort, Descending
	No equivalent

Table A.3 Formatting toolbar

Version 5.0	*Version 4.0*
	Options, Toolbars
	Options, Toolbars
	Options, Toolbars
	Draw Toolbar, Colour tool
	Options, Toolbars
	Options, Toolbars
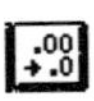	Options, Toolbars
	Options, Toolbars

Index